FIBROMYALGIA AND OTHER CHRONIC PAINFUL CONDITIONS

SECOND EDITION

FIBROMYALGIA AND OTHER CHRONIC PAINFUL CONDITIONS

SECOND EDITION

The Patient's Guide And Survival Manual
For Obtaining Proper And Effective
Medical Care

Jeffrey B. Loomer M.D.
Board Certified Rheumatologist

For information address:
Mystery Doc Publishing LLC
P.O. Box 36662
Tucson, AZ, 85704-6662

mysterydocpublishing@gmail.com

ISBN: 0984920730
ISBN-13: 9780984920730

Library of Congress Control Number: 2013912199
Jeffrey B. Loomer, M. D.

Printed in the United States of America
For information regarding special discounts for bulk book purchases, please contact Mystery Doc Publishing LLC @ mysterydocpublishing@gmail.com

Contents

I want to thank my patients, for without them this book could not have been written.

Disclaimer

It should be strictly understood that the information in this book is not intended for the reader to take it upon themselves to medically manage their own or anyone else's medical condition. Under no circumstances should any person take a medication which has not been prescribed to them by a licensed health professional, nor should anyone modify their specific medication regimen without the approval of their healthcare provider. This could cause serious bodily injury, including death. The reader should share the information in this book with their healthcare provider as to promote a positive and effective resource base for better communication and direction regarding the management of fibromyalgia and other chronic painful conditions.

Foreword

All of the information in this book is strictly the opinion of Jeffrey B. Loomer, M.D. This book is based on my personal experience of treating thousands of patients over a period of greater than twenty years. The practice of medicine is an inexact art. Qualified experts in all fields of medicine certainly may have differences of opinion, which are reflected in the way they practice medicine.

The purpose of this book is to reach out to all the people who suffer from fibromyalgia and chronic pain. I believe this is an area of medicine which is underserved. Ironically, there are millions of people in the United States and throughout the world, who on a daily basis, have to deal with these conditions. It is my true belief that nobody should have to suffer with chronic pain. The medical community has the capacity to treat these people. I find it amazing that there is such disconnect between the medical communities' ability to treat fibromyalgia and chronic pain and the lack of attention these patients are given.

I believe that throughout the years (having managed thousands of these patients successfully), that I have developed a sensible and effective way to treat these patients with cost effective medications. I have, in a positive way, changed the lives of thousands of people.

It cannot be overstressed; all of the information in this book is presented with the intention of having the reader communicate with their healthcare provider who is responsible for the medical management of their patients. Under no circumstances should any person take it upon themselves to either self-medicate or self-adjust any medication.

This is very dangerous and could result in serious bodily injury and possibly death.

This is not a "how-to" book. It is about information, which will empower the patient regarding taking the appropriate measures to put them in the best position to obtain effective medical care for the management of fibromyalgia and chronic pain.

Believing that the information in this book will be helpful to the reader, I feel I have presented worthwhile information in a novel and unique way which I have not seen in print elsewhere. I have taken over twenty years of personal medical practice experience, and created a book where patients and healthcare providers can become effective partners, and begin a productive and meaningful journey to address and manage fibromyalgia and other chronic painful conditions.

Introduction

Medicine has come such a long way since the time of Hippocrates, the father of medicine (460-375 BC). Over the past 100 years, medical knowledge has grown exponentially; yet, it is ironic that we are only just at the dawn of accepting and understanding a condition that has been with us throughout the ages. Historically, fibromyalgia has been given little recognition let alone validation by the medical community. I have been treating patients with fibromyalgia for over 20 years. I first became acquainted with this condition in 1990, when I was in the first year of my Rheumatology Fellowship at Dartmouth. I had just finished my three-year Internship and Residency training in Internal Medicine. During those tough three years, I was exposed to a vast array of medical conditions; ranging from minor ailments that were addressed in the outpatient clinic setting, to complex medical diseases, many which required management in the intensive care unit. Would you believe, after four years of medical school and three years of post-graduate training in Internal Medicine I never heard of fibromyalgia!

In my opinion, this exemplifies why physicians know very little about fibromyalgia; there has been little opportunity regarding formal training of this condition in medical school and post-graduate medical training programs. I often have wondered how this apparently prevalent condition has "fallen through the cracks" for so many years. I do have a theory about this phenomenon. First, medical students simply are not educated on fibromyalgia because historically there have been few experts in this field. As you already can see we are not off to a good start where, after four years of medical school, the knowledge that a young doctor possesses about fibromyalgia is only minimal at best.

Second is Internship and Residency. For young physicians, who choose to go into fields of medicine, other than Internal Medicine and Family Practice, the potential for these doctors to gain practical knowledge regarding fibromyalgia diminishes with each passing year. For those doctors, who take the plunge into Internal Medicine and Family Practice, it is extremely unlikely they will see a fibromyalgia patient in the hospital, unless they are involved with a patient who is being worked up in the ER or briefly admitted to the medical unit for unexplained pain. These patients quickly are ruled in or ruled out for more serious acute medical conditions. When it is determined these patients are not in acute medical danger, they often are classified as having fibromyalgia, as they are shown out the door of the hospital. Discharge instructions will tell these patients to follow-up with their primary care providers in a week or so.

The primary care providers do not know what to do with these patients. Many are branded as hypochondriacs and malingerers. If these patients are lucky, they may get a referral to see a rheumatologist, but they may have to wait a few months until an appointment becomes available. Many rheumatologists will not accept patients with the diagnosis of fibromyalgia. At this point, given this scenario, it is not looking very promising for patients with fibromyalgia. However, this is the reality of the situation. If you have been keeping track of the years, you are looking at a well-intended physician, who after four years of medical school and three years of Internship and Residency training (seven years in total), who may have virtually no knowledge, let alone experience, in treating fibromyalgia and that is a scary thought! By the way, after a doctor completes the hospital training program, it is quite possible one of the first few patients who walk into the physician's office will have fibromyalgia; the patient who was sent home from the ER the previous week! This begins the start of a long relationship of mutual frustration between the physician and patient. I really do believe this represents the life cycle of the fibromyalgia patient and the medical community.

By now, you are probably wondering if there is anyone out there who can help people (you) with this condition. The answer is "yes," but it will not be easy. This is my reason for writing this book. Physicians need to be educated about this condition. Patients with fibromyalgia need to be embraced. The present disabling life cycle of fibromyalgia needs to be broken. I know I am not the only rheumatologist or medical physician who has been treating fibromyalgia patients for many years. I know what I have learned from my patients and I am thankful to them for that. I have treated several thousand patients with fibromyalgia and other chronic painful conditions, and the vast majority of them have done quite well. Let us read on and see where you stand with these conditions, and see where you can begin your journey to liberate yourself from pain.

one

What Exactly Is Fibromyalgia?

This certainly appears to be a simple question, but in fact, the answer is quite complex. I often have looked at other people's definitions of this condition. Textbooks say one thing, not much, while self-proclaimed authorities, many of them non-physicians, have written books, and of course there is the Internet, where if it is "on-line" it must be true. On occasion, while strolling through Barnes & Noble, I would thumb through the section of books on fibromyalgia, whose numbers seem to be growing annually, and I have yet to come across a book that really delves into the therapeutic management of this condition. How can one expect a nutritionist or chiropractor or psychologist (just some of those who have authored books on fibromyalgia) to be an expert on the management of fibromyalgia when they are not physicians? Most physicians do not know much about fibromyalgia, but at least they can write prescriptions for treating this condition. There may be a few patients with fibromyalgia who can derive benefit from a holistic approach towards the treatment of their condition, but they are few and far between. I am going to cut to the chase on this issue; the vast majority of people with fibromyalgia need to be on a patient-specific medication regimen to effectively control their symptoms, but I have not seen much written about the specific medication regimens that are necessary to effectively treat fibromyalgia.

There may be several reasons for this. I believe that even in well-established medical communities in large urban and suburban regions, there are only at best a handful of doctors who know how to treat fibromyalgia. If we concentrate on just the physicians who treat fibromyalgia, the ones who really know what they are doing, you will begin to understand that these are unique practitioners; their patients and referring physicians are well aware of this fact. These are physicians, who for years, have been thinking and practicing medicine, in a good way, outside of the box.

Before the summer of 2007, there were no FDA (Food and Drug Administration) approved medications for the management of fibromyalgia. At the time of the writing of the second edition of this book (as with the first edition), there are still only three medications that are specifically approved by the FDA for the treatment of fibromyalgia. It is important to note that these three medications have been on the market for years, but the FDA had approved them for the treatment of other conditions. I will discuss these medications and others later in the book. I have been prescribing these medications and many others for some time for the management of fibromyalgia. [Note: When a medication has an FDA approval for the treatment of a specific condition, and the physician chooses to prescribe that medication for another condition, this is known as "off-label" prescribing of the medication.]

Ironically, in my opinion, there are plenty of effective medications on the market (brand names and generics) to effectively treat fibromyalgia. I have been having significant success treating my fibromyalgia patients with medications that are already on the market, some of which have been around for decades. In order to successfully treat this condition, the physician has to know what to look for and how to clinically approach the patient suspected of having fibromyalgia.

Patients are frequently referred to me because of "chronic pain." These may be individuals who for years have been dealing, most unsuccessfully, with chronic discomfort. The ways in which these patients have been managed by the referring physician varies greatly. It is amazing and sad how people can be managed ineffectively for years. I always wonder one of two things: why these physicians did not refer these patients out sooner; or why these patients did not, on their own, seek out more effective management?

In reality, the answer to this question is rather complex, and in most cases, no one is to blame. It can be quite frustrating for the general physician to manage patients with chronic painful conditions; many are uncomfortable treating these patients. If a doctor is to be effective, in managing patients with chronic painful conditions, they have to be comfortable, particularly in the prescribing of narcotics. There are plenty of patients who are, in fact, appropriate candidates for the prescribing of narcotics. In my opinion, if a physician, for whatever reason, refuses to incorporate the judicious use of narcotics in their practice, they will be ineffective in managing chronic pain in a fair number of patients who fall into this category.

How does a physician begin to develop a productive working relationship with the patient with chronic pain? It does not take long during the initial visit with a new doctor to get a sense where this new relationship is going. The attitude of both parties (physician and patient) is extremely important during the first visit encounter. A doctor, who is comfortable treating patients with chronic painful conditions, will not feel intimidated when a new patient comes to their office complaining of chronic discomfort with years of prescribed narcotic usage. Sometimes a patient on a complex pain management regimen actually will discharge their primary care physician, and seek help from a different primary care physician. The problem, in this situation, is the new primary care physician may be uncomfortable with prescribing opioids (narcotics), and the patient is right back where they started. Often, doctor offices have signs posted in the waiting room stating they do not prescribe narcotics. They tell the patients that they will manage all of their other conditions and write prescriptions for their other non-pain management medications. The only good thing for the patient in this situation is that these doctors tell their patients up-front they do not manage chronic pain, and they usually have a pain specialist to whom they will refer them.

My approach, to the patient who comes to my office complaining of chronic pain, is quite simple. I need to spend at least 50 minutes with a new patient. I want to review the records the patient has brought with them. Patients will sometimes get upset if their records were not sent to my office ahead of time. Patients usually know what tests were done and their results. I am often quite effective with making a diagnosis on the basis of taking a good history from the patient followed by a careful physical examination. Personally, I feel it is important for the doctor to obtain the history from the patient, and it goes without saying that the doctor should perform the physical examination.

In order to effectively manage the patient, with a chronic painful condition, the clinician has to determine the etiology (cause and origin) of the pain. Not all painful conditions are fibromyalgia, but patients with chronic painful conditions often have fibromyalgia. To determine if someone has fibromyalgia, the physician has to have a good understanding of what to look for. So, here is the million dollar question (which due to inflation, a struggling economy, and after taxes is really worth about half a million dollars).

What is fibromyalgia? The answer is rather straight-forward. Fibromyalgia is a syndrome. What is a syndrome? A syndrome is a collection of clinical features which as a whole defines a medical condition. Now that you know the definition of a syndrome you can begin to understand, and possibly identify, this condition in yourself; however, do not take it upon yourself to start diagnosing your family and friends. It is alright for a patient to have an understanding of a condition before going to a doctor. Just remember, you will not be an instant expert, and keep in mind a competent physician, during the course of an initial evaluation, will be considering other diagnoses too. I often have patients who either are referred to me, by their primary care provider or come on their own, telling me they think they have fibromyalgia, and they are usually right!

The most common scenario, regarding the fibromyalgia patient, is they are referred to me with the presumption of another diagnosis, such as, rheumatoid arthritis or lupus; the patient will say to me their blood work showed one of these two conditions, and I was going to treat it. This is a perfect example of a referring physician innocently missing the boat. An abnormal blood test certainly does not make a diagnosis. A positive rheumatoid factor (one of the blood tests used to diagnose rheumatoid arthritis) does not necessarily mean a patient has rheumatoid arthritis. A positive ANA (antinuclear antibody), a test used to diagnose lupus and other connective tissue diseases, does not mean a patient has lupus. The results of these tests can certainly mislead the practitioner who ordered them, not to mention scaring the patient.

It may take several months for a new patient to get an appointment to see a rheumatologist, and during that time they are worrying about a condition they really do not have. To make things worse, for the last several weeks, they also may have been on the Internet learning all about "their new condition" including both accurate and inaccurate information. Now, my job has the added complexity of deprogramming these patients and explaining to them what they really have. My favorite situation is when the primary care physician tells their patient they have a connective tissue disorder (such as, rheumatoid arthritis, lupus, or another diagnosis that falls under my field of expertise), and the patient chooses to embrace an inaccurate diagnosis by their primary care physician after I have told them they do not have that condition! Now, they think that I do not know what I am talking about!

At the end of the day, fibromyalgia is a clinical diagnosis. There are no abnormal blood studies or specific radiographic (x-ray) findings that establish a diagnosis of fibromyalgia. Fibromyalgia is not an inflammatory condition. I will say it again (this is a very important concept), the diagnosis of fibromyalgia is made on a clinical basis. Complicating the picture is the fact that fibromyalgia often co-exists with other medical conditions, and other conditions can have clinical features consistent with fibromyalgia, more about this later.

What is the constellation of historical and clinical features that add up to make the diagnosis of the fibromyalgia syndrome? The most common feature, in patients with fibromyalgia, is their inability to obtain a restful night of sleep. One of the first questions I will ask a new patient is about their quality of sleep. How do you sleep at night? Do you have difficulty in getting to sleep, staying asleep, or a combination of the two? The vast majority, of fibromyalgia patients, will respond by telling me they sleep poorly. It is interesting to note how many times patients tell me that this conversation never came up with their primary care provider. Some patients will tell me they sleep well. This, however, should not be the end of the line in questioning the patient suspected of having fibromyalgia.

The next important question, that should be asked, is about the "quality" of the sleep process. Sleep quality is a key feature in identifying, understanding, and treating patients with fibromyalgia. The usual response to the sleep quality question is these patients feel exhausted when they wake up. I often am told by patients they sleep only for a few hours at a time. It certainly is not difficult to understand these people would be exhausted in the morning since they are not getting a good night's sleep.

What about the patient who tells me they sleep 10-12 hours a night? The same sleep quality questions have to be asked. Sleeping 10-12 hours a night does not mean a person will be rested in the morning. Feeling rested in the morning and having full energy to meet the challenges of the day depends on the "quality" of sleep. Six hours of good quality sleep is more beneficial than 10-12 hours of poor quality sleep. This initial line of questioning occurs in the first few minutes of sitting down with the new patient. Just on this basis, of how the sleep quality questions are answered, quickly clues me into the patient who likely will have fibromyalgia.

When discussing the sleep quality issue with patients, I like to use the electric power tool analogy. Let us just say you are a carpenter and use a rechargeable power tool throughout the day. At the end of the day the battery charge will be low, therefore, it has to be recharged so it will be able to be functional the next day (recharge the battery overnight). Now, just for a moment, consider yourself to be a power tool that needs to be recharged at the end of the day. Going to bed is like climbing into a big electric charger, it should supply you with enough energy capacity by the morning to propel you through the day. This should be the normal cycle, more or less. If the power source to the carpenter's power tool is faulty and a continuous full battery charge is not accomplished by the morning, the tool will run out of energy halfway through the day. Without the power tool functioning, the carpenter cannot accomplish any further meaningful work for that day. There really is not much difference between the functional capacity of people and a rechargeable power tool; they both need a stored energy source to be fully functional. If a person wakes up exhausted after a night of sleep, regardless of the number of hours of sleep, that person will not have the proper "recharge" to meaningfully get through the day. If you are not rested when you get out of bed, how are you going to feel a few hours into your day, let alone by the end of the day?

The poor sleep pattern process is a fundamental problem I have recognized in thousands of patients whom I have treated with fibromyalgia. Successful identification and management of this process is the initial step to treating fibromyalgia. Based on my experience, with treating this condition for over two decades, I almost consider fibromyalgia to be a sleep disorder. I make this statement on the consistent observation that in general, these patients have poor sleep patterns and many, for the most part, improve when the poor sleep pattern is addressed and successfully treated. Keep in mind, not all people with sleep problems have fibromyalgia. Other medical conditions can cause disruption of the sleep pattern. Some people do not sleep well because of a condition called sleep apnea. In this condition, people will actually stop breathing for a few seconds and then they wake up. They often are not even aware this process is taking place. I frequently will ask the sleeping partner, if present during the evaluation, if they notice this abnormal sleep process. The sleep apnea process may be associated with snoring, so this is also an important question to ask. One myth is that sleep apnea only occurs in the obese individual. This is not true. Thin lean people certainly can suffer from sleep apnea. If this condition is suspected, the patient needs to be referred to a sleep study lab for evaluation.

Patients with sleep apnea often have features consistent with fibromyalgia. Usually, if sleep apnea is identified, and appropriate treatment is initiated, the fibromyalgia symptoms often resolve. A sleep study is quite painless. The patient packs an overnight bag and reports to the sleep lab in the evening (many labs are open seven days a week). Electrodes are hooked up to the head, heart, and a device is placed at the end of one finger to measure the amount of oxygen that is present in the bloodstream. Remember, this really is a non-painful study. (Though by the time the patient is all hooked up they look like the average patient in an intensive care unit!) This would be a good time to bring a digital camera and snap a few pictures; make up your own story and distribute them to family and friends. (I never said I was normal folks!) There is also a closed circuit visual monitor for the technicians to observe the patient's activity as they sleep. The study monitors the patient until the next morning. If the person displays episodes of not breathing, during the night, associated with brief periods of waking, and a lowering of the blood oxygen level, this would identify sleep apnea.

The treatment is quite simple. A pressurized oxygen mask is then placed over the patient's face, and they are observed for further activity. The vast majority of patients identified with sleep apnea have an immediate and dramatic response to the oxygen mask treatment; this apparatus is called a C-PAP (Continuous Positive Airway Pressure) machine, and is obviously available for home use. You do not need all the other stuff from the sleep study facility, just the C-PAP machine (insurance should cover this piece of equipment). I thought it was important to discuss sleep apnea and give the reader some insight into this condition, its evaluation, and treatment because physicians often overlook this important cause of insomnia. One of the reasons for writing this book was to empower patients with accurate and appropriate medical information they can discuss with their physician. There is no reason why a well-informed patient cannot make suggestions to their healthcare provider; noting this will need to be done in an artful friendly manner as to not irritate the practitioner.

Now that we have established that a poor sleep process is a fundamental driving force for the development of fibromyalgia, we need to examine the consequences of this problem. Patients with fibromyalgia also experience extreme fatigue. This is one feature the patient always will describe to the healthcare provider; this symptom is not to be overlooked! Well, when you think about it, one would expect the patient with fibromyalgia to be fatigued. After all, they are not sleeping properly. How can someone expect to be rested in the morning if they are not getting a good night's sleep? Let us take the equation one step further, building on the concept that a poor sleep pattern leads to waking up feeling very fatigued and not rested, most patients with fibromyalgia complain of aching all over, all the time. If this information is not volunteered by the patient, I am going to enquire about this. It is important for me to get a good understanding about the patient's "pain." Is it the muscles or the joints, or are both painful? How long has this been going on? What is the nature of the pain (dull, sharp, constant, intermittent)? What makes it worse; what makes it better; is there associated swelling of the joints; what time of the day are these pains at their worst or at their best? Patients often tell me that their joints swell, but subsequent examination usually reveals no evidence of swelling. This is not to say that patients are intentionally lying to me, it is just that their "perception" is different than what is actually going on. The description of joint swelling would alert me to carefully consider an inflammatory condition, and if truly identified on physical exam, would lead me to work up the patient for one of several arthritic conditions depending on other historical and clinical findings. Remember once again, fibromyalgia is not an inflammatory condition so swelling should not be present in a patient with fibromyalgia, except in situations where fibromyalgia and inflammatory conditions coexist. I often see this in my practice, but let us not complicate the fundamentals of fibromyalgia at this time. I will touch upon this concept later in the book.

It is certainly possible for a patient to experience swelling of the joints, which can last for several hours in the morning. It is important to keep in mind that if swelling is really occurring, this is not a feature of fibromyalgia and represents another process. I have to make clinical decisions on the basis of what people tell me and what I observe on physical examination. When a person tells me their joints swell the first question I immediately ask is whether their joints are "presently" swollen. If they tell me their fingers are presently swollen and my examination reveals no swelling, it is unlikely that an underlying inflammatory condition is present. On the other hand, if the patient tells me the joints swell for three to four hours in the morning, and I am evaluating them at three in the afternoon and joint swelling is not identified on examination; I am certainly going to consider an inflammatory condition. The investigative studies for this patient will be different than a patient suspected of having only "primary fibromyalgia" (fibromyalgia not attributed to another underlying condition). This will be discussed in more detail later.

Headaches are another common feature that patients with fibromyalgia experience. I often am told by my patients that they have been experiencing headaches from several months to several years. Many of these patients have been to see a neurologist, and unfortunately have not been helped with the use of various migraine medications. I have observed that many of my patients with fibromyalgia associated headaches experience significant relief once their fibromyalgia is under control. The treatment of fibromyalgia headache is often not simple, meaning it may be necessary to use a combination of medications to achieve the desired effect. This is actually a basic concept to the overall approach of treating fibromyalgia. In any event, the topic of headaches should come up during the initial visit. Sometimes patients will not mention headache unless I bring it up. Remember, fibromyalgia is a constellation of symptoms, and it is during the initial visit that I am trying to get an understanding of which symptoms a patient is experiencing, so that I am able to even consider a diagnosis of fibromyalgia.

Irritable bowel is another symptom patients with fibromyalgia often experience. This is a gastrointestinal process which can have several different presentations. Some patients have diarrhea; others may complain of constipation; and others may have a combination of diarrhea alternating with constipation. Keep in mind, all gastrointestinal disturbances, in the setting of a patient with fibromyalgia, cannot be assumed necessarily to be irritable bowel. When reviewing the gastrointestinal system, there are a number of questions that need to be asked. Examination is a key component, and sometimes the picture can be confusing. Irritable bowel can certainly coexist with other gastrointestinal abnormal processes. It will be up to your healthcare provider to determine whether additional gastrointestinal investigations are warranted. Further studies could possibly include blood work, x-rays, a barium study, CT and MRI scanning, nuclear scanning, and quite often the involvement of a gastroenterologist who has the ability to directly visualize the upper and lower gastrointestinal tracts through the use of an endoscope, often referred to as upper and lower endoscopies.

Once again, fibromyalgia is not an inflammatory process, so gastrointestinal disturbances strictly related to fibromyalgia should not be associated with inflammation of the gastrointestinal tract. There are several conditions of an inflammatory nature which can affect the gastrointestinal tract, which may coexist in a patient with irritable bowel, which will need to be sorted out by the healthcare provider. Sometimes a diagnosis of irritable bowel is established only after an extensive gastrointestinal work-up proves to be negative. This often is quite frustrating for both patient and physician when extensive testing is negative. However, it is important to remember even a negative test is information. A normal colonoscopy tells you a colon cancer is not present, and at least in that visualized portion of the colon, an inflammatory gastrointestinal condition, such as, ulcerative colitis or Crohn's disease are not present. Inflammatory, malignant, infectious, and autoimmune conditions often have to be ruled out before a diagnosis of irritable bowel can be determined, unfortunately, after a very lengthy and expensive negative work-up.

Memory and concentration are also frequently an issue in the fibromyalgia patient. Again, these are features which are not readily volunteered by the patient. It certainly makes sense that if a person has a poor non-restful night of sleep their mental functioning is not at full capacity the next day. The term "fibro fog" has been used to describe an altered state of cognitive function which many patients with fibromyalgia experience. This process may be manifested by an inability to focus on simple conversation, poor short-term memory, confusion and difficulty with even simple mathematic calculations. I have had patients who on occasion cannot even remember their own telephone numbers, home address and zip codes. Correction of the sleep pattern is usually what it takes to improve this problem. Once again, the complexity of addressing and successfully treating fibromyalgia depends on sorting out and identifying one medical process from another.

Memory and concentration difficulties can be caused by a vast array of medical conditions. Depression and anxiety are quite common in the general population affecting people of all ages. Other causes of memory and concentration difficulties can be due to the natural aging process; dementia and Alzheimer's (in elderly individuals), seizure disorders, vitamin deficiencies, central nervous system diseases due to inflammatory, infectious and malignant conditions, as well as, recent and remote head trauma. This is by no means a complete list, but just a brief example to remind the reader for every symptom fibromyalgia patients experience, there is a differential diagnosis that needs to be considered. It may be necessary for the patient to see a neurologist for an appropriate work-up which can be costly and time consuming (brain imaging studies, special blood studies and sometimes a lumbar puncture (a procedure in which, following anesthetizing (numbing) of the area, a thin, long needle is inserted between the space of two of the lower lumbar vertebrae and then spinal fluid is withdrawn for analysis). Neurologists do this procedure on a frequent basis and complications are minimal.

Tingling and numbness in the hands, feet, or both are also common features patients with fibromyalgia experience. As a general rule, I am more likely to attribute this complaint to fibromyalgia if the neurologic features are symmetric (occurring on both sides) and are affecting the hands and feet. If the symptoms are occurring in just a hand, foot, or an entire limb, another cause of this symptom needs to be investigated, identified and appropriately treated. Compression of a nerve needs to be determined, especially if the neurologic symptoms are focal (localized to one specific area). A nerve being compressed at the neck or lower back can cause tingling, numbness and even a burning sensation, as well as, increased sensitivity to touch at a site remote to where the actual pathology is taking place. Neurologic symptoms in the hand can be generated from a process in the neck (even without associated neck pain). Tingling and numbness in a leg or foot can be coming from a problem located at the lower back (even in the absence of lower back pain).

Sometimes these patients are referred to me by the neurologist after they have determined their neurologic symptoms are just part of an overall picture of fibromyalgia. I certainly do not want to give the reader the impression that the presence of symmetric abnormal neurologic processes point only towards fibromyalgia. Degenerative arthritic processes involving the cervical spine (neck) and lumbar spine (lower back), often can be associated with symmetric neurologic processes. Diabetics often get a symmetric neuropathy which on description can be compatible with the neurologic symptoms experienced by fibromyalgia patients. Carpal tunnel often affects both sides. There is a whole differential diagnosis for patients with neurologic symptoms. Certain medications can be associated with neurologic side effects, some of which may not be reversible, as in the case of certain chemotherapies used for the treatment of various cancers. Other causes of neuropathies can be due to autoimmune diseases, vitamin deficiencies, various central nervous system disorders, and one very big one needs to be mentioned: alcoholism. This is once again not a complete list, but another example of how there is a differential diagnosis for all the symptoms that patients with fibromyalgia experience.

Chest pain is also a symptom which is often described by the fibromyalgia patient. When a patient complains of chest pain the physician has to take this symptom very seriously. Cardiac disease has to be considered; especially in the older patient, but young people can also experience cardiac disease. Many of these patients have been sent to an urgent care, emergency room, or cardiologist only to have a negative cardiac work-up. These patients are then given the label of "non-cardiac" chest pain. The complete work-up for chest pain entails certain blood studies; an EKG (a recording of the electric activity of the heart), echocardiogram (an ultrasound of the heart), cardiac exercise treadmill (the EKG is recorded while on the treadmill and an echocardiogram is also done during this procedure) and cardiac nuclear imaging (a procedure in which a substance is injected into the vein and is taken up by the heart tissue and the heart activity is monitored and recorded). Sometimes it is necessary to perform a cardiac catheterization (a procedure in which a catheter is placed in an artery at the groin region and is then advanced up to the heart). A special dye is then injected through the catheter into the coronary vessels (blood vessels of the heart), and this enables the cardiologist to determine if any of these vessels are clogged, which could possibly explain the reason for the chest pain.

There are a host of other symptoms patients with fibromyalgia often experience. Shortness of breath is sometimes described. An underlying lung condition needs to be considered and ruled out. Many patients (especially the elderly) have lung conditions such as COPD (chronic obstructive pulmonary disease); this usually exists in present or prior smokers. Many patients, both young and old, have asthma and seasonal allergies. All pulmonary conditions can have episodes of exacerbation, and these are symptoms that may be described to the physician during the initial evaluation of a patient with fibromyalgia.

Some patients complain of bladder irritability. Bladder problems are certainly common in the elderly population (men and women). Urinary stress incontinence is frequently observed in both elderly and not so elderly women; this would not be a feature of fibromyalgia. Having the sensation of needing to urinate, but otherwise emptying the bladder normally, may certainly be a fibromyalgia associated symptom, but other pathologic conditions need to be ruled out. Medications, such as antihistamines (allergy medications) can affect the bladder and cause urinary retention. Bladder symptoms, associated with fibromyalgia (in my experience), are not as common as the other symptoms I have already described.

Psychiatric illness also is quite common and often coexists in the patient with fibromyalgia. Depression is usually associated with insomnia, and by now you know the consequences of insomnia. One question often asked is: "Which came first, the depression or the fibromyalgia?" Sometimes the answer is clear. Patients often tell me they have had depression for years, and on further questioning it appears the fibromyalgia symptoms developed much later. Sometimes patients tell me they are depressed because of the symptoms of fibromyalgia. Many fibromyalgia patients whom I have treated have depression, and for many of them I do believe this is secondary to the fibromyalgia process; this really does make sense; how can a person in chronic pain be happy? I will discuss my approach to treating this situation as well as fibromyalgia in general in a later chapter.

In closing, CHAPTER ONE: "What Exactly Is Fibromyalgia?" I think the first thing that we need to establish is that it is not a condition where we can be totally "exact." We can, however, understand this is a chronic condition often associated with a constellation of symptoms which are not inflammatory in nature. It is a real condition, whereby, there will be no abnormal laboratory findings, and the diagnosis will depend on an awareness of this disease entity, historical and physical findings, and the absence of findings that would point to another medical condition. But most important, fibromyalgia is a condition that affects millions of people in this country (and I suspect throughout the world), knows no ethnic or socioeconomic boundaries and for the majority of people (at least in my over 20 years of experience) there are effective and available medications for the management of fibromyalgia and other chronic painful conditions.

Additionally, one of the reasons for writing this book was to empower patients with accurate and appropriate medical information they can discuss with their physician. There is no reason why a well-informed patient cannot contribute medical information and even make suggestions to their healthcare provider. Remember, successful treatment of fibromyalgia and any other painful condition for that matter, will hinge strongly on a good patient-physician relationship.

The reader will not be an expert after reading this book, but will possess sound knowledge and a better understanding of the fibromyalgia syndrome, allowing for better use of the allocated time for the office visit with the healthcare provider. This should also provide a better understanding as to whether the most appropriate healthcare provider, who can most effectively help you, is being seen, or if following the initial visit it is recognized that care may need to be sought elsewhere. The reader will know what type of information is important to tell the practitioner, and be able to engage in a meaningful discussion about fibromyalgia in a sensible way. It is often a long road in just getting to the right place.

The journey to effective treatment, even by a well-seasoned practitioner, who embraces fibromyalgia, can be quite frustrating. During the initial visit it is important not to get into a long discussion about things that really do not relate to the problem at hand as this may put off the healthcare provider, and exhaust the allocated time for the office visit, thereby losing the opportunity to convey important medical information.

I think we are off to a good start. We will continue to keep building on this knowledge as we forge ahead. Stay with me; the journey has begun, and we will keep it at a pace which makes sense. Knowledge empowers, now let us move forward together.

two

Living With A Chronic Painful Condition

There are a lot of people out there who live and suffer with pain on a daily basis. I see these people in my office every day, and I am sure there are considerable numbers of people who suffer in silence. Whatever the cause of the "chronic pain," at this point, it is not going away of its own accord. By virtue of the fact that we call the pain "chronic," there should be an understanding it is here to stay. This, however, does not mean you have to be suffering chronically.

How do you know if your problem is chronic? By the time people usually get to see me, their pain is chronic, and this is not because it took so long to get an appointment. Painful injuries and processes which tend to resolve over a few weeks to a few months fall under the category of "acute;" there is an endpoint to the pain; and the process is expected to heal. We have all experienced this type of pain: an uncomplicated broken bone, post-surgical pain, bursitis, tendonitis, sprains and strains. These conditions tend to be self-limiting, as they do get better on their own or with the help of a medication that is not expected to be used on an ongoing basis. Some self-limiting conditions may take months or even up to a year to settle down. It could take up to a year for a back surgery to feel good. Unfortunately, even with the most skilled of surgeons, back surgeries are often not helpful and sometimes the patient is even worse after the surgery. A hip or knee replacement may take up to a year to feel like it has always been there. The point is, self-limiting pain, from a sense of time, can have a chronic component.

In my practice, I see a lot of patients who suffer from chronic pain. I am not referring just to my fibromyalgia population. Many of these patients may have secondary fibromyalgia. [Note: This refers to fibromyalgia that has developed as a secondary process to an underlying painful condition.] One of the most common types of patients, who I see, is a person who suffers from chronic lower back pain. There are many causes of chronic spinal pain. Aside from the lower back, many suffer from upper back pain and less often from mid-back pain.

As we advance this discussion on chronic pain, it is important to quickly review some pertinent points regarding the body's anatomy. The spine extends from the base of the skull to the lower region of the tail bone. The medical terminology for the upper portion of the spine is the cervical region. This consists of seven cervical vertebrae and from the top to the bottom they are numbered: C1-C7; the C stands for cervical. Moving downwards, along the spine, is the thoracic region (thoracic spine). There are twelve thoracic vertebrae and heading from north to south they are numbered: T1-T12. Moving further, south, are the lumbar vertebrae, totaling five in number: numbered as L1-L5 (where L5 is at the lowest portion). The short bit of bone below L5 is the sacrum, commonly known as the tail bone. The spine is full of vertebrae and a whole lot of other structures (disks, ligaments, blood vessels, closely associated muscles, and do not forget about the spinal cord and all the nerves exiting through passages created by one vertebrae in close proximity to another).

In order to feel pain, you have to have a nervous system. The central nervous system is the brain. It is the brain that processes all types of stimuli which is fed to it from the peripheral nervous system, that is, nerve tissue that resides outside of the brain. As a general rule, nerve tissue (nerves) runs parallel and in conjunction with blood vessels (arteries and veins). This is why when you cut yourself, not only do you bleed, but it hurts too! There is a reason for this short "basic" course in anatomy. To understand pain, you need to have some understanding of the nervous system. You will begin to see how pathology (abnormal anatomy) can lead to pain. In order to effectively treat pain, the physician/healthcare provider has to know what is wrong before an attempt can be made to try to effectively address the problem.

Keep in mind, throughout the course of this book; I just want to remind the reader that my writings are based on my observations and practical treatment of thousands of patients since 1990. After so many years, you tend to see the same problem over and over and hopefully have gained good practical knowledge and success from the experience of treating all of those patients. [Note: In no way, do I want to minimize the suffering of chronic back pain; I embrace people with this problem.] The fundamental concept, of patients with chronic pain, is that they will need medication therapy. The specific types of medications will be discussed later in the book. Of course, it is not my mission to give everyone, who walks out of my office, a prescription or two or three, etc. I can tell you from my experience, for the average person with a true chronic painful condition, who walks through my door, conservative modalities are not going to cut it. Besides, most of these patients have been there and done that, and are at a point where their primary physician does not know what to do with them. Some come to me on their own, because they are in constant pain, and their healthcare provider has told them essentially, there is nothing more they can do for them.

Aside from painful spinal conditions, people have chronic pain for a variety of reasons. I often manage patients with chronic pain in a limb. This can be caused from an injury, such as, from a motor vehicle accident. Most doctors do not want to be involved with injuries resulting from accidents because there is often litigation in the process, and several months or even years later the physician may be drawn into the legal process (depositions, short and long-term disability claim forms and possible in-court testimonials).

Often diabetics have limb pain because of peripheral neuropathy and this can be quite debilitating. I also see a lot of patients, who just experience chronic generalized pain, which is not fibromyalgia. This is extremely difficult to treat because of the subjective nature of the pain. Usually, there is nothing focal (localized) with regard to their pain. They usually have normal blood work and all investigative studies, such as CT and MRI scans, are all normal. Sometimes, more invasive tests are done and here, too, the findings are normal. Is it possible to have chronic generalized pain with normal studies and a normal exam? The answer is "yes," but good luck with getting appropriate treatment when you walk into most doctors' offices with this set of medical features.

Of course, there are a small percentage of patients, who do present with vague symptoms, with normal lab and clinical findings and the answer is not a medication. Some patients complain of pain, but further digging, into the family circumstances, reveal a family dynamic is at the basis of the visit. I sometimes have to point this out to the patient and family member or members who are present; often with a mixed response from the parties, who are present. Sometimes, I will tell a patient, on their first visit, I am not able to help them. In this case, it is usually because they need to be seeing someone else (counselor or psychiatrist). I am not telling these people there is nothing wrong (something is always wrong), it is just that I am not the most appropriate person, to treat them, for their ailment.

Chronic Pain

Who gets chronic pain? Anyone can. My medical practice has been and continues to be devoted to the adult population (18 years and older); it should be understood that the comments in this book are directed to the adult population. Pain is non-denominational and presents without discrimination. I treat patients with chronic pain ranging from eighteen years old and upwards. These are people who have chronic painful conditions, which just are not going to go away, without some type of medical intervention.

Keep in mind, the term "medical intervention" does not mean necessarily the use of prescription or, for that matter, non-prescription medication. Medical intervention can involve counseling, qualified medical manual manipulation, ultrasound treatment, physical therapy (which includes all of their therapeutic modalities: ultrasound, massage, traction, heat and ice applications and most important, the instruction on how to properly perform physical exercises).

There are many components to the disposition of people living with chronic pain; the source of the pain makes no difference. Some people suffer from localized pain, while others from more nondescript generalized discomfort. The common thread, with these people, especially by the time they get to my office for evaluation and treatment, is that there is often an element of depression (regardless of which came first; the pain followed by depression or depression followed by pain). There tends to be anger, sometimes directed at me, during the first few minutes of the initial evaluation. Keep in mind that it would be in your best interest to be civilized with the doctor who holds the greatest chance of helping you. You do not want that visit to end with the doctor telling you that you would be better suited to see someone else, because of incompatibility issues. These patients often feel hopeless, helpless and abandoned by the medical community. On the initial visit with me, I listen closely, review available records, perform a pertinent physical examination and most importantly, I validate their suffering. I tell them, I truly want to help them with their pain, which really is true, and I will work diligently with them to improve the quality of their lives. Believe it or not, making significant improvements in treating chronic pain is not difficult if you are an experienced doctor, who knows how to treat chronic pain.

People with chronic pain are actually quite patient, considering what they have been dealing with, often for years. These patients understand their pain will not go away overnight; or perhaps ever, if at all. What they are looking for is an honest attempt to help alleviate the "degree" of suffering. Chronic pain management is all about "relative" levels of improvement. By the time many patients get to my office, they feel the visit will be an exercise in futility and I can understand why. Many have been to chronic pain clinics and specialists, but unfortunately, have not been helped; in spite of what I would consider, on the basis of their medical history, a good attempt. Some of the failures, I have observed, are both physician and patient related. Every doctor treats pain differently. For the most part, chronic pain patients are best managed by a practitioner, who embraces these types of patients. Specifically, I am not saying chronic pain only can be effectively managed by a "pain specialist."

Who is a pain specialist? Classically speaking, when your healthcare provider sends you to pain management, you will be seeing an anesthesiologist; bear with me on this for a moment. Although classically trained in anesthesiology, with which you are probably more familiar (putting people to sleep for surgery and then waking them up), these physicians now have practices that are based in combination in the office and procedure room. These are the doctors who perform medical and diagnostic procedures under fluoroscopy.

Fluoroscopy is a medical procedure, where the patient is placed in a medical procedure room; which consists of a medical table, for the patient to lie on, usually on their stomach. The area where the procedure is to be performed is cleaned, so the site where the needle will be introduced will be sterile. Next to the procedure table is an x-ray machine, which enables the physician, usually, but not always, an anesthesiologist, to view the desired region of the spine. This enables the physician to place a needle precisely into the region where the medication is to be delivered. Before the needle is inserted, the area where the needle is going to be introduced is infiltrated (injected) with a local anesthetic such as Lidocaine or Marcaine. When this procedure is performed, by a skilled clinician, the patient usually only feels the anesthetic being administered, this really is not too bad. The discomfort only lasts for a few seconds. The rest of the procedure, from the standpoint of the patient, usually is quite painless. In fact, it usually takes more time to prep the patient (getting the patient in place for the procedure; getting the equipment and support technicians in place; and preparing a sterile area where the needle is inserted) than to do the procedure. The medication which is injected is a type of steroid (a very safe and potent anti-inflammatory). [Note: This type of steroid is different than the type you hear about in the news where athletes inject themselves to bulk up their muscles.]

The clinical symptoms and the findings on an MRI study, of the area of interest, will dictate where and what structure or structures will be injected. The anatomy of the spine is complex, and depending on where the pathology exists will dictate where the medication is to be delivered. Anyone, who has one of these procedures, has to have had an MRI study of the region of interest. It is going to be this study, which may identify the exact location of the problem. Also, the age of the MRI has to be taken into consideration. If a patient has chronic lower back or neck pain, and an MRI was done six months ago, it may be necessary to order a new MRI before a procedure is performed, especially, if there has been significant progression of symptoms or the presentation of new symptoms.

Neck Pain

I often have an elderly patient who presents with the complaint of neck pain. The first thing I want to know is: how long the problem has persisted? Was this a gradual process? This, would at least initially, lead me to think this is a degenerative process (wear and tear between the vertebrae). There is a cartilage disk between each of the vertebrae; think of this disk as a cushion or shock absorber. Unfortunately, body parts wear with time, some faster than others, and this is a body component that often wears down as we get older. Certain traumas can certainly create or predispose the patient to an accelerated degenerative disk process. As this process progresses, regardless of the etiology, neck pain develops. [Note: This process is usually associated with decreased neck range of motion.] Sometimes this process also can be associated with pain, weakness and/or numbness of an upper extremity, if there is associated cervical (neck) nerve involvement. This is a clinical situation which can be addressed in several different ways or in a combination of ways.

Let us take a closer look at what is going on, and why the clinical symptoms are experienced by the patient. The degenerative (or traumatic) process is creating abnormal mechanics of the normal neck physiology. Alignment of the neck is very important. Any process, that affects alignment, is going to have an impact on all of the associated neck structures. There is a lot of stuff (bones, muscles, nerves, blood vessels and parts of organ systems) which passes through the neck region. Under normal situations, these neighboring structures communicate and coordinate with each other in a peaceful manner. Let us use, as our example, degenerative cervical disk disease. As the disk progressively wears away, this is potentially going to have a cascading effect on the basic integrity of a normal neck complex. I am sure you can picture the impact that a worn out cervical disk can have on related neck structures. As the disk begins to wear away, this results in less space between the adjacent vertebrae. As the vertebrae get closer and closer together, this is going to have an impact on normal neck alignment. This process alone is enough to create neck pain just on the basis of neck muscle spasm, without any direct irritation of the cervical nerves.

Spasm usually is associated with decreased neck range of motion. There will be a natural guarding process (which will limit normal neck range of motion) to avoid exacerbating the existing painful neck process. As a further continued consequence, the neck muscles become weak and this too will contribute to an ongoing process of neck pain. The head is a heavy part of the body and it takes strong neck muscles for proper support.

It is often the case, that the degenerative disk process also may be associated with an arthritic process. This can create further misalignment of the vertebrae; in addition to this structural abnormal process, cervical nerves can be irritated or compressed. When this process presents, the patient usually experiences pain, weakness, or numbness, or any of these in combination. This is a more serious situation than just pain. These are features associated with nerve compression and need to be addressed to avoid permanent neurologic (nerve) damage. When this process develops acutely, especially if there has been a trauma, a herniated (slipped) disk has to be considered, evaluated and managed without delay. With an acute neck injury, professional medical personnel should be contacted immediately (911). Do not manipulate an acute neck injury! This can cause severe injury to the spinal cord and can result in permanent injury or even death.

Physical therapy, as a mode of treatment, can be very effective for patients with chronic cervical pain. What is the physical therapist supposed to do? When I send a patient to the physical therapist for management of cervical pain, I want the physical therapist to do several things. Because of the chronic nature of the neck pain and the associated consequences of this chronic painful process, I want the patient to be taught an exercise strengthening program. This will help the patient to strengthen the neck muscles; remember cervical muscle strength is important to support the head. Additionally, I want the patient to improve their cervical range of motion.

One simple example, of poor cervical range of motion, is how it can negatively impact safety associated with driving a motor vehicle.

We already have driver blind spots and rear view visibility varies from time-to-time. Elderly patients are often criticized for their driving skills. Decreased cervical range of motion is an important issue for decreased driving skills in the elderly; poor vision and decreased reaction time are also other factors, which contribute to diminished vehicle operator skills in the elderly.

In order to accomplish my request with the physical therapist, he/she will also need to do additional therapeutic modalities, which helps alleviate pain at the time of the physical therapy sessions. These modalities may include: ice and/or heat application, massage, traction, electrical stimulation (TENS unit), or ultrasound treatments. These therapeutic modalities often are used in combination. Some of these treatments actually may exacerbate the discomfort; the therapist will know how to develop a protocol that best fits each individual. These are qualified professionals, who have gone through years of special schooling to do what they do. I have never met a physical therapist who I did not like; they are good people, and they have a lot to offer those who suffer with chronic pain. It is amazing how many general practitioners underutilize the physical therapist. You should mention this mode of therapy, to your healthcare provider, if they do not mention it first.

Most patients, following a series of physical therapy sessions, come back to my office and report to me, they have had good success (keeping in mind that the interpretation of "good" and "success" will mean different things to different people). For the sake of discussion and direction, I am going to sub-classify the patients with neck pain who have gone through physical therapy into different groups. The first will be the group of patients who tells me they feel great, no pain, back to baseline, and they will make a "prn" (as needed) follow-up appointment, if something new comes up. Obviously, these people are quite happy; they feel better, and as their treating physician, I take pleasure in the fact their problem has resolved and this was accomplished without the use of medication. I get to see these patients as needed; unusual scenarios in my practice since the majority of conditions, I treat are chronic; these patients need to be monitored with varying degrees of frequency.

The second category of patients, are those who have gone to physical therapy, and have had a partial response. Here, too, there will be varying degrees of intervention. So what happens with these patients? Now we need to consider a medication regimen. Many of these patients already may be taking one or more medications for their neck pain (not to mention other medications), which already may be on board for the treatment of one or more medical conditions. Keep in mind, although physical therapy may not have taken away all the pain, the patient may have derived "some" benefit which is of significant value. Pain is a relative process. People, who have been living with chronic pain, are used to suffering. Any type of incremental reduction, of pain, is always welcomed by these patients, especially when they know I am on the journey with them, and we are traveling in the right direction.

Back Pain

Let us address back pain. There is a lot of it out there. I see several people a day with this ailment. The spectrum of patients, with back pain, who I see in my office on a daily basis, can range from an acute strain or spasm to chronic unremitting pain, which has been present for decades. I get to see all the failed back surgeries, and the subclass of patients who truly have a surgical problem, but because of other coexisting medical problems, the surgeons feel surgical intervention would be too risky. What happens to all of these categories of back pain sufferers who come to my office? Is there hope for any of them? Does the degree of pathology limit the success of treating this problem? What about the patient who has been to another rheumatologist or anesthesiologist, who has been attempting pain management unsuccessfully? Does this mean that I cannot help them? Does this mean that there is no hope? Here is my answer: every patient needs to be properly evaluated. I need to know what the problem is; what investigative studies have or have not been done; and what modes of treatment have been offered, tried, or refused, and the degree of success or failure that has been met with treatment attempts.

Sometimes, I see patients, who actually have been offered very minimal therapy. Other times, it is my opinion, that a good attempt at treatment has been made, but perhaps the wrong medications were selected, or improper dosing (either too much or not enough) of medication has been prescribed. I also see patients, who are treated with inappropriate medications, or there may be duplications of medication classes. A patient, for example, may be taking two different NSAIDs, such as ibuprofen and naproxen sodium (either in prescription strength or over-the-counter dosages). There are also patients, who are seeing more than one doctor, and are getting medications from each of these doctors. These patients either knowingly or unknowingly do not tell each doctor about all of the medications they are taking. I have several patients, who have chronic pain, which I co-manage with another pain specialist, such as, an anesthesiologist. In this situation, I usually prescribe the pain medications and the anesthesiologist does the fluoroscopic procedures; epidural blocks and other procedure room oriented treatment modalities such as the placement of dorsal column stimulators. [Note: The dorsal column stimulator is a device which is implanted in the lower back to stimulate the spinal cord with electrical impulses in patients with severe back pain. This device is certainly not for everyone with back pain.]

I have some patients, who have a dorsal column stimulator, and it can be quite helpful for lower back pain management; however, it may not be effective for some people. Before this device is implanted there is a test which is performed on the patient. What happens is that the patient is brought into a procedure room where there is a fluoroscope next to the procedure table. The fluoroscope is an x-ray machine which allows the doctor to visualize the spine so that when they are doing a back or neck procedure (such as an epidural) they are able to see where they are placing the needle; so they know exactly where they are going.

In the case of testing to see if a dorsal column stimulator will be effective, the doctor places wires through the skin into the spinal cord region where the pain is originating. The fluoroscope is used to make sure that the wires are guided into the right place. [Note: As painful as this may sound it really is not.] The patient is given local anesthetic to the region where the wires are to be inserted. This is the most painful part of the procedure. The patient will feel a sting for a few seconds and then the area is numb. From this point onward there should be no further discomfort when the wires are inserted. Then the doctor will pass an electric current through the wires. If the dorsal column stimulator is going to be successful, the patient will immediately feel relief of the pain when the electric current is turned on. The hope is that the electrical stimulation will override the back pain and give the patient relief. If this works the doctor then takes the wires out, and at another scheduled visit the dorsal column stimulator is implanted. You definitely want to make sure that it is going to work before going through the procedure and expense which is involved with implanting the stimulator.

Lower back pain is quite complex. Management usually involves multiple modalities: medications, physical therapy and invasive proce-dures, either minor (such as, an epidural injection) or major (which can involve a minor or major neurosurgical operation). Back pain can be either localized or generalized, depending on the exact region of involvement. Causes of back pain also vary. Older patients are more likely to develop back pain because of a degenerative process, such as, wear and tear arthritis. The history usually will be enough to lead the clinician to this diagnosis, but x-rays should be done for confirma-tion. Other imaging studies, such as, an MRI, are sometimes needed to make a more definitive diagnosis. It is not uncommon for clinical symptoms (back pain) and imaging studies not to correlate. A person could be experiencing significant back pain with associated numbness going down one or both legs and x-rays and MRI's are not showing anything abnormal. I often see this in my practice. If a patient has acute or chronic back pain and nothing abnormal is identified, by an imaging study, does that mean nothing is really wrong with the patient? The answer to that question is "NO." Is the patient not telling the truth? It is a possibility.

Lower back pain is a problem I see at least a few times a day. Who gets lower back pain? All types of people: young, old, male and female. My practice is limited to patients eighteen years and older and I manage back pain in the full range of these patients. [Note: Most patients whom I treat with back pain have it because of degenerative arthritis, wear and tear arthritis.] Men and women are affected equally. The age group for this set of patients usually begins in their forties, yes their forties! Many of these patients look well in every respect, but the back pain limits their quality of life. Why is it a person, in their forties, who has no history of back trauma and has not abused their body in any way, develops this problem? I can only explain this on the basis of my observations throughout the years in treating patients with this problem. [Note: I have been encountering these issues several times a day since 1990.]

Does obesity play a major role in the development of back pain? I treat a large number of obese patients who do not have back pain. However, one certainly cannot underscore the impact obesity has, on not only the spine, but the whole body. I would like to comment on the age old statement that many obese patients, with back pain, have probably heard at one point in their life from a healthcare provider, "If you can find a way to lose 40-60 pounds, your back pain will get better." To be quite honest, I have told this to patients in the past. These patients almost never would come close to losing 10 pounds, let alone 40-60 pounds. They would return to my office a few months later (weighing the same), still complaining of back pain. My response was always the same, "Your back is not going to feel better until you lose the weight." I really did think that was the answer.

Weight loss is a very difficult thing to do, and even more importantly to maintain. To be successful, with permanent weight reduction, several barriers have to be broken. Dietary changes are a must, which is not so easy, especially for extended periods of time. Exercise is important, as is proper "quality rest." There is a large psychological component to the barrier of weight reduction. First, you have to believe that significant weight reduction can be accomplished. Second, aside from mapping out a dietary plan and exercise program, one needs to identify and modify the "non-hunger cues" for eating. What does this mean? Well, think about this for a moment. We do a lot of eating when we really are not hungry. We probably eat more food a day, away from the dining room table, then when we are seated at it. Of course, I do realize that our lives are complicated: kids, work, school and a host of other issues that add up to the fact that we need more than 24 hours in a day to accomplish what needs to be done. We often eat a lot of fast foods; where everything has to be supersized. I am not trying to be cynical or critical here (I am as guilty in indulging as the next person). My point is, if we think about it, we have more control over our weight than we think we do.

Returning to obesity and back pain; I have made a rather interesting observation in a small subset of patients. These are the patients, with chronic lower back pain, who have had either a gastric bypass or the lap band procedures. The vast majority, of these patients, have not derived significant reduction of their back pain, after losing as much as 150 pounds. Please keep in mind; this is only my observation, in a very small number of patients. However, I must say this: these patients have been quite pleased with their weight loss.

Aside from the obvious weight loss, these patients have made significant strides in other aspects of their medical state of well-being. Such parameters as blood pressure, diabetes, hypercholesterolemia, fatigue, depression and self-image derive secondary gain from these procedures. Several of these patients have had to spend their life savings to pay for these procedures, but all of them have told me that it was worth it. Unfortunately, many health plans do not cover these procedures as medical benefits. In my opinion, aside from the patient benefits, which are a given, it would be more cost-effective for the insurance company to foot the bill for this procedure up-front. It is going to cost a lot more than the gastric procedures, down the line, when the insurance company has to shell out money for such "covered" procedures as: knee, hip and back surgeries, and let us not forget about managing cardiac disease, such as, cardiac stents and bypass procedures. Throw in diabetes and all of the multitude of potential complications of this condition, not to mention a host of other medical factors, which are affected by obesity, and the cost skyrockets over that of one of the gastric procedures. Obesity will have an impact on mortality.

I think the rationale, on the part of the insurance companies, hinges on the fact that most people do not have the same health plan five years down the line. If, this is truly the case, from the economic standpoint of the insurance company, there may be the attitude of, "Why should we foot the up-front costs of this procedure, when down the line, they will not be our responsibility and the next insurance company benefits from our expenditure." Keep in mind, I am not saying this is what they are thinking, but it does make sense from an uncaring, cold and distanced economic standpoint.

It also should be noted, with regard to these gastric procedures, they should not be viewed lightly. At least, in the case of the bypass procedure, forever there will be a change in the way one eats. Supplements have to be taken; it is a life-altering procedure in many ways. Also, as with any procedure, there are risks of serious complications. One would need to get the full story from the surgeon specifically trained in these procedures. There is also the cosmetic effect of significant weight reduction. Often, after these procedures, there is excess skin which hangs from the abdomen, arms and legs. This leads to the subsequent need for cosmetic surgery to address this issue. I did have one patient, where the insurance company actually paid for the gastric procedure, but the patient was on their own when it came to the cosmetic component, following the surgical procedure.

From a joint standpoint, it has been my observation that significant weight reduction, from these gastric procedures, tends to give greater relief of peripheral joint pain (feet, ankles, knees and hips) and to a much lesser degree, to the lower back. Remember, this is only my observation in a limited number of patients in my practice. One explanation, to this phenomenon, may be due to the fact that the arthritic damage has taken place already, keeping in mind, that significant weight reduction will not change the already damaged architecture of the lower spine. One could argue the weight reduction may have an impact on the rate of further progression of degenerative changes. This may already be a moot point, since the patient is already in pain.

However, pain is relative. Less pain is better, more pain is worse. Everyone has their own level of what would be considered acceptable versus unacceptable pain.

Back pain can have many presentations. The most common cause of back pain that presents to my office is due to degenerative arthritis; a wearing down process that affects the intervertebral disks (the structure that separates one vertebra from the other). Think of this structure as a spacer between the bones of the vertebral spine. The natural course of events, with the vertebral disk, is this structure wears down as we get older. [Note: This is not a problem that only occurs in older people. The rate of the degenerative process varies between people.] There are genetic factors, but also non-genetic factors, which will have an impact on the degenerative process of the disk structure. Trauma can potentially initiate the degenerative disk process, which, in any given person, may not have begun until decades later. Think of injuries from motor vehicle accidents, sports related injuries and certain genetic or acquired metabolic disorders that can have a negative impact on the integrity of the disk structure. When the integrity of the disk structure is compromised this can lead to a host of clinical presentations of back pain.

The fundamental concept, with regard to the spine, is this unit of multiple interconnected and interrelated structures has to work in concert with each other, and when this does not happen, the seed is planted for a potentially ever growing painful process which can branch out in several directions. We feel pain because we have a peripheral and central nervous system. Under normal conditions, the nervous system is responsible for many important functions of the body. We have voluntary movements (walking, running, standing, sitting and reaching); you get the point. Neurologic function, such as breathing, would be an example of involuntary movements. Of course, you can hold your breath, but when not thinking about breathing, we just do it; think of breathing during sleep.

The brain (the central nervous system) interprets information that is delivered to it, via nerve fiber connections from outside of the brain, the peripheral nervous system. When you touch something hot or cold, it is the nerve fibers of the peripheral nervous system that sends a message to the brain (the central nervous system). The brain interprets the significance of the signal and an immediate action is taken: drop a hot object, turn on the cold water faucet to offset the hot water, etc.

In the case of back pain, there is a problem affecting nerve fibers along the spinal region, which then sends a signal to the brain; this is interpreted as a painful process. So, your senses should tell you that back pain that is spinal, in origin, is coming from some process that is interfering with the structural relationship between the vertebrae, tendons, ligaments, muscles and blood vessels. Any structure, which causes pressure to be exerted onto any portion of a nerve fiber, in the region of the lower back, will in turn deliver this sensory information to the brain. So, if a disk is pushing on the spinal cord, this will not only cause the sensation of back pain (often incapacitating), but there also may be functional abnormality associated with this process (pain radiating down the leg; weakness in the lower extremity, on the side where the disk is being impinged; or possible numbness in the same distribution). Arthritic changes, involving the vertebrae, often create a situation where nerves are being impinged, which leads to a chronic painful situation. Of course, any trauma to the spine can create an immediate disruption to the integrity of this tightly knit community of interrelated structures, and hence, the beginning of a painful process that can be lifelong.

Having a good understanding of microanatomy, particularly the distributions by which nerves exit the spinal cord, can give an astute clinician a good idea, at which level of the spinal column, the injury has occurred. The specific abnormality in many cases needs to be further identified by one of several types of imaging studies, such as, an MRI, CT, x-ray, or contrast medium study. These studies often are performed in combination with an electro diagnostic study (a nerve conduction study/electromyography). This is a diagnostic procedure, which usually is performed by a neurologist. Electrodes are attached to either one or several limbs: electrical shocks and/or mild needle probing is done along the limb in question, to evaluate the presence and location of where a spinal abnormal process may be originating. The results, of this type of study certainly, may hinge on several variables. Unfortunately, these tests are not always accurate. I often send people with unilateral or bilateral limb numbness for this study, and the test may come back normal, however, the patient still is complaining of a numb limb! The test may come back normal, but try telling that to the patient, who now is no nearer to a diagnosis, but in addition to their ongoing problem, they just paid a co-pay and to obtain the study may have missed a half-day of work!

Treatment and Management

Physical Therapy

The value of physical therapy must never be underrated. I some-times have to enter into heavy negotiations, with some of my patients, when recommending physical therapy as a primary mode of treatment. There is the initial resistance since a prescription is not being written, except for the one I hand the patient to give to the physical therapist. This mode of therapy is wrongly perceived as inferior to a prescription medication, and this is just going to be a waste of time and money (co-pays, deductibles, cost of travel and time away from work).

Factors will impact everyone differently depending on their own personal situation. A retired person with good insurance coverage, which I would define as being responsible only for a nominal co-pay, if any, may certainly embrace the concept. I ask my patients what their insurance plans cover and do not cover. They usually know, and if they do not, I either have my staff make the inquiry or advise the patient to contact their healthcare company to find out the specifics of their benefits. Do not forget, every healthcare insurance program has a cus-tomer service number you can call to get the information for which you are looking. The number is usually on the back of the insurance card. Remember, be nice on the phone; you want the person on the other end to get it right. There is less incentive for the person on the other end of the line to accurately help you, if you are angry, shout-ing, or using profanity. If you feel you are not getting anywhere, you certainly have the right to ask to speak to a customer service manager, but do it in a nice way. It can be done successfully; I do it all the time with various issues with which I frequently deal.

The value of physical therapy is certainly a modality of treatment that should be available and utilized in the appropriate setting. Let us look at some real life common examples of patients, I have sent for physical therapy. I see a great deal of lower back and cervical problems. Before I can consider any therapy, I comprehensively have to evaluate the patient. This entails a complete medical history and appropriate physical examination. In this history, I also want to focus on what has or has not been done to treat the complaint; but also, what has been done to evaluate the problem. Sometimes patients come to me after having all the right studies done to evaluate the problem; other times, the work-up can range from no diagnostic studies to an incomplete work-up. Sometimes no studies are indicated. This depends on the presentation, location of pain, and duration of symptoms with regard to treatment or lack of treatment response.

Throughout the years, I have sent countless numbers of patients to physical therapy for a host of various musculoskeletal complaints. I have had many success stories, especially, where people have had chronic neck pain. They became pain-free after a course of physical therapy, and most importantly they continued with a regular regimen of exercises they did on a daily basis at home. The physical therapist usually wants to see the patient initially two to three times a week for several weeks. This is important and do not try to scale back the visits. Be committed to the physical therapist. Your dividends will be big. After the initial protocol, the visits will be less frequent; this will be mutually determined between the patient and the therapist. The long-term plan is to empower the patient to be able to maintain a daily program that will continue to provide benefits for years to come.

One important note that would be very helpful to tell the health-care provider, who will be writing the prescription for the physical therapist, is how the request should be written. For example, the prescription should request, "Cervical spine muscle strengthening program with range of motion exercises." Another important bit of information that needs to go on the prescription to the physical therapist is, "any modality prn (as needed)." This is very important to the patient and is quite helpful to the requesting healthcare provider. This will allow the physical therapist to do whatever is appropriate. If this "blanket permission" is not included on the prescription certain modalities may not be rendered. By not specifically writing this, on the prescription, it may cause extra work for the practitioner because the physical therapist will be calling asking for permission to do these therapeutic modalities. This will involve, from the practitioner's end, having to pull your medical chart; taking the phone call from the therapist or calling them back at a later time, hopefully not too late because the patient is probably at the physical therapist's office waiting for the approval. Approval will then involve another prescription, requesting the extra therapeutic modalities, which were left off of the initial prescription request.

Getting the physical therapy prescription request right from the onset is very important. First, the patient will get what is needed without further delays. Second, there will be less frustration on the part of the physical therapist, since multiple requests for additional services will be avoided. Finally, there will ultimately be less additional work for the healthcare provider, who is making the request for the physical therapy. Get the initial prescription right and everyone will be happy.

It should be noted that various insurance companies have different rules about physical therapy coverage. It is not uncommon for me to get a second request, from the physical therapist, to submit another prescription for additional visits. I always comply with the physical therapist's requests. I have had many patients, who initially were skeptics, when I suggested physical therapy for non-medication management of neck pain and other areas of pain. These people go on to become the biggest proponents of physical therapy. I prescribe many medications for a lot of different conditions as the majority of my medical practice is chronic pain management. If I can avoid using medications I certainly want to go that route. Physical therapy has allowed me to use less numbers and amounts of medications in various patients I treat for chronic pain.

Management

The purpose of this book is to offer hope and more importantly "help," to people suffering from fibromyalgia and other chronic painful conditions; not to identify a drug seeking individual. As already mentioned, I do not believe that a pure drug seeker wants to read this book. [Note: For the rest of this book, as well as, the preceding pages, my intention is to reach out to the true sufferers, out there, who are looking for help.] All of the case examples are real, the pain is real, and there are not any other hidden agendas that need to be exposed. I would like to point out to the reader; although, I must be constantly vigilant for the drug seekers, the insurance scammers and disability wannabes, most people who walk through my office "do not" have a hidden agenda. I need to evaluate, on a continual basis, who needs what, how much and/or for how long. Chronic pain management has logistical challenges for the prescribing physician.

Medical records need clear documentation with appropriate time interval office visits with strict control and tabulation of narcotics. Many doctors are concerned about the potential for regulatory scrutiny, and fear losing their license, to practice medicine, in association with the prescribing of narcotics. This is why some offices have signs posted stating that the physicians in their office, "do not prescribe narcotics." Some of these doctors' concerns also may have an impact on the types and doses of narcotics that they dispense. I often assume the narcotic management of patients, who are referred to me by other physicians. These physicians are certainly well-intended for their patients; they may even have them on a narcotic along with one or several non-narcotic medications that are commonly used for pain management. Sometimes the problem may be that the physician is not prescribing an adequate dose of the medication.

All people respond differently to medications. Certainly, there may not be any correlation to the size of a patient and the dose of a medication necessary to effectively address someone's pain. I have treated little old ladies in their eighties, whose pain is not controlled without high doses of combination narcotics; and 250 pound middle-aged men who develop mental status changes on even the lowest dose, of what I would consider to be a mild narcotic. The fact of the matter is, everyone is unique, and medication regimens have to be "custom tailored." I often tell my patients, when it comes to pain management this is not "off-the-rack" medication shopping. Your couture may not be custom tailored, but in my office your medication regimen will be! This is why I can see ten different people, in one day, who have the same problem (back pain), and I can show you ten different medication regimens.

What determines who gets what? That is actually an easy answer. I need to know what medications have been taken in the past. What has worked and what has not worked? Are there any allergies I need to worry about? By the way, if a patient tells me they did have an allergic reaction to a medication, I always make it a point to have the patient tell me exactly about the nature of the reaction. If a person tells me the medication caused a stomach ache; that is not an allergy, it is intolerance. Keep in mind; I still am not going to give that medication to the patient. However, if a patient tells me they took one anti-inflammatory and developed a severe life threatening reaction that landed them in the ICU (intensive care unit) not only will I not be giving the person that medication, but I likely will not be prescribing them a similar drug from that medication class.

I also need to know about the doses of medication that were taken in the past. If a patient tells me, a particular medication that was previously taken was not effective; it may be because an inadequate dose of the medication was prescribed. I have had countless patients who were deemed non-responders to medications, only to find success when prior used medications were reintroduced at a higher dose. Sometimes, I will prescribe combinations of medications that were once deemed failures, when administered as single agents, and now have great success. As a general rule, combination therapy can give better results than if each drug were used as a single agent at different times. Combination therapy also affords the ability of prescribing less doses of each medication because of the synergistic (additive) effect between the two (or more) medications. Also, patient finances come into play, when I have to create an appropriate medication regimen. Insurance co-pays vary from policy to policy and company to company.

What about patients who do not have insurance coverage or medication coverage? What about the person who has coverage, but who takes so many medications the cost burden of just one or two more medications cannot be handled? What about the psychological effect of adding even more medications to a person already on a host of other medications for other medical conditions? Let us not minimize the effect, of the introduction of chronic pain medication, to the patient who never has taken medication before on a regular basis.

Other factors that play into the decision making process when prescribing medications include: an awareness of other ongoing medical issues, for which the patient is being treated; as well as, other medications that are already prescribed; this may limit some of the available medication options. If a person also has kidney disease and/or a history of gastrointestinal bleeding; or if they are on blood thinners, an anti-inflammatory needs to be avoided. Age may have an impact on medication prescribing. As you can see, there are a lot of factors that need to be taken into consideration when developing an appropriate pain management medication regimen.

PLEASE READ THIS NEXT PARARGRAPH
VERY CAREFULLY!!!!!

I need to mention specifically something at this point in time. Please understand the information, about these medications I have previously discussed or will be discussing in the following pages, is for informational use only. With regard to the medical management of fibromyalgia and other chronic painful conditions, discussed in this book, this is not a "how-to" book. It specifically is "not" my intention to enable the reader to self-medicate or to experiment. Many of these medications are commonly prescribed to treat various conditions. If you already have these medications in your medicine cabinet, at home or may have relatives or friends that take these medications and you feel you can start taking these medications on your own, perish the thought!!! Do not under any circumstance ever take a medication, on your own, which has not been specifically prescribed to you by either a doctor or qualified healthcare provider. You have to understand, there may be contraindications for you to take certain medications, which only your healthcare provider would know. Not all medications can be safely taken together. As innocent as you may think it might be, I am specifically telling you "not" to self-prescribe as this really could create a deadly situation. When it comes to medications, which I mention in this book, it is for informational purposes only; feel free to discuss the content of this book with your healthcare provider and do not take it upon yourself to self-medicate!!

three

Medical Management Of Fibromyalgia And Chronic Pain

It has been my experience, the vast majority of patients with fibromyalgia need to be on some form of a medication regimen. The presenting clinical features will dictate the required medication formula. This is where the true art of managing this condition comes into play. My experience, in treating these patients, has taught me, there is no specific medication which will help all patients and address the myriad of symptoms, which may vary between individual patients. I can show you several different patients I have deemed to have fibromyalgia, and their presenting clinical features can be so diverse, one would not expect all of them to be classified as having the same diagnosis. You can begin to imagine how confusing this must be to the patients, let alone the primary healthcare provider, who likely, has no formal training with this condition. Even the so-called "experts" on fibromyalgia, whoever they are, have different opinions about this condition, and their medication prescribing patterns are reflective of this phenomenon. [Note: There is no cookbook recipe for the management of fibromyalgia; there never has been and probably never will.]

Certain aspects of medicine are quite cut and dry. A urinary tract infection needs to be treated with an antibiotic; the majority will be effectively managed with a course of a conventional antibiotic. [Note: There are always exceptions to the simple rules.] However, this is not the case when treating fibromyalgia and other chronic painful conditions. In order to effectively treat fibromyalgia, the clinician has to have considerable understanding of medication classes; what good and bad potentials each medication holds; and how they, not only interact in combination, but also, how they interact with other medications, prescribed by other practitioners, for other conditions. This is one reason why it is so important that a medication review is done at the beginning of each visit. The healthcare provider needs to know about all medications from all providers.

Another important concept, the patient should be aware of and often overlooked by the healthcare provider, is to determine if the patient is also taking over-the-counter medications. A few examples are the patient who takes a prescribed anti-inflammatory and takes it upon themselves to take an over-the-counter ibuprofen (Motrin) or naproxen sodium (Aleve); usually motivated by advertisements. What they do not realize, and how would they, is these medications should not be taken together because of potentially serious (life threatening) effects on various internal organs, such as, the liver, kidney and gastrointestinal systems.

People on blood thinners need to avoid non-steroidal anti-inflammatory drugs (NSAIDs), even at the low dose, over-the-counter strengths, as this could cause potential life threatening bleeding. A nose bleed can be controlled with packing gauze and direct pressure; a gastrointestinal bleed can be deadly for obvious reasons. [Note: As I am writing this chapter, I am typing away at 35,000 feet, on a Southwest Airlines flight. Anyone developing a significant gastrointestinal bleed in this situation will probably die. What am I supposed to do, if a voice over the loud speaker asks, "Is there a doctor on the plane?"]

Remember, what I am about to outline is my opinion about the medications that should be used for the management of fibromyalgia. This is based on over 20 years of direct patient experiences. Yes, my patients have been my teachers. I was willing to take the journey with them and to take the roads less traveled; they were not even roads, just uncharted open terrain; sometimes a thick jungle! O.K. Who am I kidding? I live in Arizona. We don't have jungle. We have desert, and a lot of cactus!!!

SECTION ONE

Tricyclic Antidepressants (The Journey Begins)

During my rheumatology fellowship at Dartmouth (1990-1992), the standard drug of choice for treating fibromyalgia was amitriptyline (Elavil). [Note: This medication is classified as a Tricyclic antidepressant.] Why would we use an antidepressant for the treatment of fibromyalgia? Were all of these patients depressed? It did seem that most of these patients did have a degree of depression. Was the fibromyalgia a manifestation of depression? Were they depressed because of the features of fibromyalgia? These were all questions I had, but nobody had the answers. [Note: Fibromyalgia patients were not seen by the attending physician, but rather my mentors would tell me, "This is an interesting patient who will be a good teaching experience for the new rheumatology fellow." It turns out, 20 plus years later, they were right, but not for the same reasons!]

Getting back to my early years of prescribing antidepressants to the fibromyalgia patient, took a bit of negotiating with the patient. Using amitriptyline as an example, this was not an FDA (Food and Drug Administration) approved medication for the management of fibromyalgia. [Note: At that time there were no medications approved for the management of fibromyalgia.] I was essentially shooting from the hip, with the use of amitriptyline; however, it was working for many of my patients. From the standpoint of a physician, it is quite unsettling when you are sailing in uncharted waters with patients, and not really having clinical resources to answer questions and to be advising treatment options. I had to impart on my patients a sense of self-confidence so they would have confidence in me. I thought I was at least moving in the right direction with my patients. If worse came to worst; I was just treating depression with a "diagnosis appropriate" medication. I was, in general, prescribing doses that were much lower than one would use for the treatment of depression and I did not believe I was hurting anyone. I began to think everyone should be on an antidepressant, and they should be added to the water supply! Soon, I was gathering information from my patients based on my prescription pattern; in my own mind this data was becoming information: my information.

Here was my first "consistent" observation about treating patients with fibromyalgia. They all want to be heard and taken seriously; and want a practitioner who is willing to work with them. By the time many of these patients came to see me, I was the end of the line of a host of consultations and dead end avenues. These people are generally desperate for help and have gone through great lengths for pain relief; some having spent thousands of dollars on every gimmick imaginable. At the end of the initial visit, I had to give people hope that "today" was the beginning of a new direction. Often, medication would not be started at the first visit; I needed to make sure that baseline blood work was in order; and there were no other medical conditions that could be presenting with fibromyalgia features. [Note: Hypothyroidism always has to be ruled out noting that hypothyroidism and fibromyalgia can co-exist in the same patient.] Medication management would usually begin at the second visit, after I had an opportunity to review baseline blood work and any additional outside medical records, when deemed necessary.

So now, the moment of truth is supposed to begin at the end of the second visit. Where do I begin to treat these patients? Well, amitriptyline was there. I now had to convince the patient I was about to put him/her on an antidepressant using a drug which was not approved for their condition (as there was none). There was not much known about their condition, and I had to get through the patient biases and stigma of using an antidepressant. Do not forget, these patients had high hopes for treatment success; after all, this was "Dartmouth Medicine," the New England medical Mecca! To close the deal with these patients, I would tell them, I realize they are not depressed, but the use of amitriptyline, although off-labeled, was the "industry standard" for treating this condition. Besides, in my mind, many of these patients were depressed, so what was the harm? This was a safe and inexpensive medication, which was helpful in many patients with fibromyalgia. After a few success stories of my own, I was beginning not only to feel comfortable with what I was doing, but I began to think I was somewhat of an authority. I was not an authority, but who could contradict my thinking, I was the one seeing all these patients.

Another early observation, in these patients, was they all had poor sleep patterns. Interestingly enough, a poor sleep pattern was a symptom that was not volunteered by the patient; I was the one who had to ask about it. It just seemed to make sense to me, if they were not sleeping well; they were not going to be rested in the morning. If that was the case, I could see how the rest of their day would fare. Our example medication (amitriptyline/Elavil) was very helpful in many of these patients for sleep. I soon began to make the connection; when these achy, fatigued patients got a restful night of sleep, they felt better. The key was providing that refreshed (restorative) sleep process. Not only, were they feeling more rested in the morning and having less difficulty getting out of bed, but non-related symptoms also improved. They were experiencing less muscle and joint pain, memory and concentration was improving, overall functional capacity improved, muscle tenderness was diminished, and they were more happy in general, and yes, they were even less depressed, too.

They were definitely happy with their progress, and of course, with me. I was quite pleased on all fronts. I could not exactly explain why they were getting better or the exact (or even non-exact) mechanism by which the amitriptyline was working, but nobody was complaining. I was beginning to feel somewhat like a fraud, but in a good way (somewhat like a Robin Hood) stealing medications from the psychiatrists (antidepressants) and giving them to the poor orphaned fibromyalgia patients. My thoughts, of fraudulent behavior, soon changed to heroism. I was a first year rheumatology fellow and I was already making a difference. Medicine is a tough field to tackle, let alone master. Even today, and more so then, you never really think you know everything you need to know. At least, with this condition of fibromyalgia, I did not feel behind the eight ball. In fact, I actually felt I was on par with understanding fibromyalgia, and possibly even ahead of most practitioners, who supposedly knew about and treated this condition. What was turning out to be a good situation for me was an even better situation for my patients. I was on a roll and they were rolling alongside of me.

I then began to feel more confidence in treating these patients. Doctors will tell you success, with regard to effectively treating patients, builds confidence. You cannot get this from a book or taking notes on it in class; you have to live the results with your patients. I still wondered how it was, that a single dose, of an antidepressant at night, was able to make many of these patients feel so much better, and most interesting, with the first dose! It is well recognized, by physicians and psychiatrists that antidepressants can take weeks, if not months, to be effective when treating depression. Often, there is a journey with getting the desired response and the right dose of an antidepressant. They are often used in combination, and the adequate response certainly does not take place overnight. How was it that many of my patients were feeling better after the first dose of amitriptyline? In many cases, their moods were also significantly improved; they would even tell me they were less depressed among other positive things, too. So, what was this telling me? Well, I soon developed the attitude, that for many of these patients, their primary problem was "not" depression.

Primary depression would not respond, so quickly, to such a low dose of an antidepressant. The amitriptyline had to be working in some other way, and it was doing it quickly. What was going on here? I deduced the following: these patients all had the common denominators of experiencing a poor sleep pattern, with a non-restorative sleep process, that is, they did not sleep well and woke up achy and fatigued. Improving their sleep "quality," more important than sleep "quantity," was making the difference. By the way, with fibromyalgia patients, it does not matter if they are in bed for 10-12 hours at night, they are still not rested with all those hours in bed; it is all about sleep "quality." In many ways, I consider fibromyalgia to be a sleep disturbance abnormality. There is a fine line with regard to calling a condition fibromyalgia versus a patient experiencing the daytime manifestations of insomnia. Their features are quite similar; perhaps they are one in the same. I am not so worried about splitting these fine hairs; my fundamental approach, to each of these conditions, fibromyalgia and insomnia, are the same. The primary initial mode of therapy should be geared to addressing the abnormal sleep pattern.

To understand how amitriptyline exerts its beneficial effect, on the fibromyalgia patient, one needs a basic and brief tutorial on the sleep cycle; in my opinion the key feature which is abnormal in the classic fibromyalgia patient. It is rather interesting to think that the underlying process, which generates widespread pain, and the host of other symptoms associated with fibromyalgia, stems from an abnormal sleep process. This concept is often confusing to the patient. They feel pain and think, or they may have been told by another healthcare provider, that fibromyalgia is an inflammatory process. They think they should be on an anti-inflammatory or even a steroid. Many patients came to me who were prescribed, in a well-intended way, narcotics for their discomfort. The key, take-home lesson is to understand that primary fibromyalgia is not an inflammatory condition; nothing is inflamed. Patients may feel like they are inflamed, but they are not. Also, blood work will not be abnormal in these patients, unless there is something else going on. There is nothing to be found on x-rays. By the time many of these patients present in my office, they have been through the mill, having had costly medical studies which were unrevealing. So, as you can see, by the time they get to me, I tell them they do not need any more studies. Many of these patients feel there are more studies to be done, and all the previous healthcare providers, and myself, are missing the boat. Then, when I tell them they need an antidepressant, their first response is to head for the door.

Let us get back to the sleep cycle and its relationship to the patient with fibromyalgia. Keeping it simple, sleep architecture is broken down into two components, REM sleep and non-REM sleep. REM stands for rapid eye movement. During the average night of healthy sleep process a person should go through 4-6 sleep cycles. We now need to focus on the non-REM cycle. This is the component of sleep associated with giving us that refreshed restorative sleep process. It is in this stage of sleep that we get recharged. Not to get too complicated, but we need to look a bit deeper into the non-REM cycle to understand, at least in my mind, where the primary problem with fibromyalgia originates. Think of the manifestation of fibromyalgia as a cascading domino effect.

All medical problems have to have an origin. Atherosclerosis (hardening of the arteries) is related to high cholesterol and or high triglycerides. Hardening of the arteries is the end result of our bodies' inability to handle lipids. To prevent the end result of high lipid levels, we want to take measures to control these levels; the approach in this situation may be through exercise, diet, medication, or a combination of all of the above. The same goes for high blood pressure and diabetes. If we can control these medical problems, we can do our best to minimize end stage consequences of these conditions. The same goes for fibromyalgia; control the primary problem and this should prevent or minimize further clinical manifestations.

Let us get back to the significance of the non-REM sleep cycle. The non-REM sleep cycle is further broken down into four stages: simply called stages one, two, three and four. Stage four, of the non-REM sleep cycle, is where the money is. It is stage four, of the non-REM sleep cycle, that is not adequately achieved in fibromyalgia patients. This has been demonstrated in sleep studies. [Note: I do not send my fibromyalgia patients for sleep studies unless I am attempting to rule out sleep apnea.] Whether this abnormality is identified on a sleep study, or not, my approach to the fibromyalgia patient is going to be the same; my first step is to stabilize the sleep pattern.

It turns out amitriptyline enhances stage four of the non-REM sleep cycle. By doing this, patients are able to get that restorative sleep process. Hence, a restful night of sleep is associated with less aching in the morning. It is this restorative sleep process which, in my opinion, makes it a dead-end for the propagation of the other features which, collectively adds up to the fibromyalgia syndrome. Better sleep is associated with better energy, more focused concentration and memory, and often time, chronic headaches are improved. When these parameters improve, patients will tell me they are less depressed and feel less anxious.

Another important feature, which is often unaddressed, is the impact chronic pain has on the patient's relationships with family members and in the workplace. Not only is it difficult for the patient to deal with pain, but it is also a challenge for the people around them. Chronic pain issues can certainly be a deal breaker in a relationship. I have seen many a marriage end because of the impact that chronic pain has had on the spouse. Chronic pain is disabling; it changes your way of life. It can alter your mood and disposition and make you behave in ways that many employers would deem unacceptable.

Up until now, I have mentioned only the antidepressant amitriptyline. This is actually the first medication I prescribed for my fibromyalgia patients; this was my starting point. What about the people who did not respond to amitriptyline or who had side effects from this medication? What was going to be my back-up drug? At first, this was a problem for me; what do I do now? The most common side effect I observed in the patients I treated with amitriptyline was dry mouth. Keep in mind, this medication can be associated with a host of potential side effects; as can every other medication on the market. If, you actually closely read the package insert of any medication, the description of "potential" side effects is enough to scare you from taking any medication. I know the specific "common" side effects that occur with every drug I prescribe. I know which drugs can and cannot be mixed and where the contraindications exist.

I make sure all concerns (the patient's and mine) are addressed before the end of the visit. If, I cannot find the answer in my PDR (Physician's Desk Reference), I will call my local pharmacy, in the presence of the patient, and discuss my concern with the pharmacist. [Note: The PDR is a reference book which lists all the prescription medications and gives a complete profile of the medication, including possible side effects.] When I prescribe a medication, I will tell the patient what side effects to look out for, knowing and stating to the patient that all medications can potentially be associated with multiple types of side effects. I specifically tell people, if they are curious about the medication and read the package insert or look it up on-line they should not be discouraged from taking the medication. Another thing, I often tell patients, is a majority of the medications I prescribe for the management of fibromyalgia and chronic pain are not FDA approved for these conditions. The medication description will not mention fibromyalgia or chronic pain; their initial thinking, after picking up the prescription, is that I do not know what I am doing; why did I prescribe them an antidepressant or an anti-seizure medication? We will talk about anti-seizure medications a little bit later.

Let me say a few words about off-labeling prescribing. There are multiple medications that are commonly used to treat medical conditions that are not specifically FDA approved for the management of that condition. In order for a medication to receive an FDA indication for the management of a specific medical condition, the drug has to have gone through very rigorous and stringent patient studies, which document safety and efficacy. The guidelines are very specific with regard to these well-controlled studies. By the time a drug reaches the market, for its specific indication, the pharmaceutical company may have spent hundreds of millions of dollars in research and development. Now, a doctor may take it upon himself/herself to give a specific medication to a patient with a condition that is not the one for which the drug is FDA approved. This is what is called off-labeling of the medication.

I will give you a commonplace example of the off-labeling of a medication that has been practiced by physicians (at least rheumatologists) for several decades. A common condition I treat is called Raynaud's. This is a condition that is characterized by cool hands and feet. Sometimes these regions will turn bluish, when exposed to cool temperatures; sometimes, even when going into their freezer for a few seconds. Ironically, I live in Tucson, Arizona, and see a fair amount of Raynaud's. You would not expect too much Raynaud's in a town where 4-5 months a year the temperature is over 100 degrees. The fact is, as warm as it may be in Arizona, most of the buildings are kept quite cool. I like to keep my office cold, a good way to monitor how well my Raynaud's patients are responding to treatment.

Raynaud's is a blood circulation problem. The cool temperature causes the peripheral small blood vessels in the hands and feet to go into spasm. The spasm causes constriction of the blood vessels, and this subsequently causes diminished blood flow. This causes the hands and feet to feel cold. The concept of treating this condition should be to relax the constricted blood vessels. One of several classes of medications, that are used to treat elevated blood pressure, is a group of medications called calcium channel blockers. These medications cause the blood vessels to relax and hence lower blood pressure. By relaxing the blood vessels, the normal flow of blood is restored in the Raynaud's patient and the symptoms subside. I often prescribe calcium channel blockers to my Raynaud's patients; this is an example of off-labeling a medication. There have been no controlled FDA studies that make calcium channel blockers an indication for the treatment of Raynaud's; it is just a well-established, commonly prescribed class of medication for Raynaud's. There are many other drugs, on the market, which have been used for decades, which are prescribed on a daily basis in an off-labeling fashion to treat common conditions.

Getting back to the alternative for amitriptyline, what was I now going to do? I really did have all my eggs in one basket. I figured if amitriptyline was working well in many of my patients, why wouldn't another antidepressant of the same class work just as well? If, that were to be the case, then I would have another 10 medications I could use instead of amitriptyline, and that is exactly what I did. I began to extrapolate the potential of other similar antidepressants. Soon, I was prescribing such tricyclic antidepressants as: doxepin, nortriptyline and desipramine, to name just a few. Yes, these medications were also working for many, but of course, not all, of my patients. Now, I had some prescribing leeway, if amitriptyline was not helpful or tolerated, I would switch to one of her "sister" drugs.

At least now, I had a sense of direction for my fibromyalgia patients. There was no doubt in my mind, the number one priority in these patients, was to stabilize and improve the sleep process. Keep in mind; this was certainly not the magic cure. Just improving the sleep quality in many of these patients was, for the most part, by no means, the end of the story. I recognized, early on in my training, as time went on, there was a lot more going on in the fibromyalgia patient than just a poor sleep process. Chronic pain certainly has an effect on a person; on their general disposition and even their personality. These components of a chronic painful condition may not change so fast once the pain is under control, if these issues are even amenable to change.

The next step is to reevaluate at the next visit; to see where the dust has settled after the initial treatment. Experience has taught me that the response, to any medication I prescribe, for the management of fibromyalgia, should have its impact with any given dose within a few days. There may initially be some side effects with the first few doses; these generally subside with continued use of the medication. It is, for this reason I will usually start with a low dose. Aside from trying to avoid potential side effects, when initiating a new medication at a low dose, I also want to use the least amount of medication, if possible; I can always raise the dose, and this is generally what I do.

As an example, when using one of the tricyclic antidepressants, such as, amitriptyline, doxepin, or desipramine, I start the patient on a ten milligram tablet and tell them to take the medication just as they are about to go to bed. I then tell them the most common side effects of the medications are dry mouth and, they may possibly wake up groggy on these medications. The grogginess usually goes away after a few doses, if not, I instruct the patients to take the medication one hour earlier. If, after one week on the medication, there has not been any significant positive changes in their overall condition (and providing there have not been any significant side effects), I tell the patient to double the dose. Keep in mind, this medication needs to be taken before going to bed. If, the patient is a shift worker and their nighttime begins at eight o'clock in the morning, and this is when they are going to sleep, this is when they need to take the medication. Remember, the concept is to improve the quality of the sleep process. So this is what is done usually after the second visit; after I have had an opportunity to review appropriate records from outside sources, and the baseline blood work I have obtained informs me there are no other conditions that explain the reasons for their symptoms. In short, treatment begins after I am convinced they do indeed have fibromyalgia; this could sometimes begin at the initial visit. As a general rule, regardless of even a previous diagnosis of fibromyalgia, I always want to make sure the diagnosis is accurate. Sometimes, I may not agree with the diagnosis, even if they supposedly were given it several years ago.

One of the key issues of treating patients with fibromyalgia and chronic pain syndromes is you really do know where you stand with pain control, with any given dose of a medication, and with any combination medication regimen after only one week. This is why, I tell my patients to make incremental dose changes after one week. If, after one week, there have not been any changes, there will not be any positive effects with continued use of the medication without either a dose or medication change. I cannot tell you how many times, I see a new patient who had been given the diagnosis of fibromyalgia and was started on a medication (for the sake of an example it really does not matter what medication was given), and told to come back for a follow-up appointment in 3-4 months. This is absolutely ridiculous, and tells me the healthcare provider does not really know much about the management of fibromyalgia or chronic pain. After I initiate a medication, I need to see the patient in two weeks to see how things are going. It is extremely rare for a patient to hit a home run on the first dose of medication. There is usually a journey of dose adjustments and combination medication therapy, which is needed to really fine-tune the patient with fibromyalgia or chronic pain. If you remember what I just said, at the end of two weeks the patient will have most likely doubled the dose of medication. This means that after one week of treatment there was a dose adjustment, and I will be seeing them one week later.

During that initial two weeks of stepwise medication treatment, things will either have happened (good or bad) or possibly no change at all. I do believe, with the initial management of fibromyalgia and chronic pain conditions, patients need to be followed every two weeks with medication adjustments being made on a weekly basis, under my instructions. A big part of the successful management, of these conditions, is the development of a good working relationship between the patient and healthcare provider. Frequent visits, early on in the management of these conditions, not only creates a strong foundation of trust between both the patient and healthcare provider (but also in my opinion), is necessary for the proper pace in which these conditions can and should be addressed. It is important, for me, to give the patients an early verbal outline as to my initial approach of medication management. I tell them it certainly could take time and several visits to make inroads with treating their condition. Certainly, I am "not" going to start them on a medication and tell them to come back in 3-4 months! Even, with just the initial visit, I make every attempt to let the patients know there is "a new sheriff in town" and I intend to do things differently and take them in a new direction; I cannot think of anyone complaining after I make this statement!

This takes us to the end of the second visit, now what? Well, that depends upon what is discussed during that visit. People with chronic pain certainly have got a lot to say. I spend a considerable amount of time with patients during the initial consultation. I need to cover a lot of ground. I take a lot of notes, and also make notes on the notes from other healthcare providers. By the end of the visit, I have an idea and plan on which path I will take the patient. That path will vary from patient to patient. This is where the art of treating fibromyalgia and chronic pain comes in; this is not going to be found in a text book. Success in treating these patients is not going to be off-the-rack; it has to be a custom fit.

The decision, as to which medication(s) I prescribe, will be based on prior medication failures and successes, clinical features, present medications that are on board: allergies, other medical conditions, contraindications, age, and in women pregnancy status. There is a great deal of information that needs to be extracted during that initial visit. I also have to ask many questions because there may be very important pieces of information the patient does not volunteer which I need to know; conversely, some patients feel it necessary to give me way too much information. Throughout the years, I have developed a way of dealing with the latter. I let patients know I do not mean to be offensive by redirecting the conversation, but I only have a certain amount of time to accomplish what I need to do for their benefit; it usually goes over well when I put it in those terms. Besides, many patients often tell me, I am quite thorough with my history taking and physical examination; I have to be to get it right! Remember, there is only so much time for the visit; make it count! Say what needs to be said, but do not be a broken record. Also, avoid non-related information. If you bring a family member or a friend to the visit, it is important for them to not ask the healthcare provider questions concerning their personal condition. If, at all possible, try not to bring small children to the appointment; if they start crying or misbehaving this will certainly not work to your advantage; it may cause the healthcare provider to lose focus or possibly cut short the visit; make the most of your visit, do your part.

The next step, at the end of the second visit, is to determine what the next adjustment should be. Although, I am concerned about addressing all of the ailments the patient with fibromyalgia is experiencing: fatigue, headaches, tenderness, irritability, depression, and difficulty with memory and concentration, the abnormal sleep process must improve before these other features are able to improve. At the second visit, my main concern is the patient's sleep quality. If, there has not been any improvement of the sleep pattern, I do not expect anything to have changed from the prior visit. So this will be my starting point at the second visit.

My first concern is whether the medication is causing any side effects. Once I have cleared that hurdle, I then focus on sleep quality. I do ask about the other symptoms, too. If, the medication is well tolerated, but has not been effective, my next step is to increase the dose. It is interesting to observe how people respond and tolerate medications differently. I have had situations where a 220 pound person has significant side effects with even the lowest dose of a medication; and a petite eighty year old patient needs to be on maximum strength dosing to achieve the desired effect. This is why I use the start low and go slow rule. There are, however, exceptions to this rule. Experience has taught me, when a patient is taking a particular class of medication, still using our prototype example of a tricyclic antidepressant (at a relatively high dose), and the decision is made to change this to another antidepressant of the same class, I will start the patient at higher doses for two specific reasons.

First, I know from experience, if I change medications and use what would be considered a starting dose of the new medication, I am not going to see the kind of positive response when using a low dose in a patient who is not on that class of medication to begin with. I realize this is not a very scientific statement, but this has been my observation. If, I low ball the dose, I am quite sure the patient is probably going to tolerate the medication, but will not derive any benefit from the low dose. I do not want to waste time at the lower dose because this is not only going to be frustrating for the patient, but they may develop the attitude the medication is going to be ineffective and they may request another medication. If this pattern continues, with low dose prescribing of a medication and little results, one runs the risk of going through many potentially good medications which were not given a good enough chance for success. It is all about the dose. I stress this to my patients. It is going to be a journey.

The second reason, I need to change out the medication with a higher than normal starting dose, is to avoid the potential for a medication withdrawal process. When I make the changes in this fashion, I have not observed withdrawal issues. So, if the patient has not derived any benefit from the medication or a partial response is obtained, that is, sleeping better, but still not great, and most importantly, not experiencing that refreshed restorative sleep process; I will increase the dose of the medication with the instruction to make another incremental dose adjustment in one week, if the medication dose is tolerated, but their symptoms have not improved. The next visit is scheduled for two weeks later. At the next visit, I will ask the patient where we stand at that time. As you can see, there is a pattern as to how I work with each individual drug. The question, from this point onward, will be how high a dosage do I go with for the initial starting drug; and where do I go with adding a second, third, fourth, and yes, even a fifth drug! The bottom line is that it is a judgment call. This will be determined by the response to the starting medication and quite frankly my gut instinct. Again, this is not very scientific, but my methods have been quite effective; you will have to believe me on this one. That is why I am able to write this in my book; this type of statement would never fly, in even the worst medical journal.

For educational purposes and the intent of moving forward, let us say a person is now taking what I would consider the maximal dose of our tricyclic example, and they are doing better, enough for me to not want to substitute this medication with another tricyclic, but not good enough to call this the end of the road; what is my next move? This will depend on the prevailing residual symptoms. I do not mean to make things complicated here, but remember I am still talking about how I was treating patients in 1990, given the available medications at that time, and my embryonic knowledge of fibromyalgia at that time. As the years passed, I developed new attitudes, opinions, and approaches to the patients with fibromyalgia and chronic pain. New medications were introduced into the market; many not specifically approved for the treatment of fibromyalgia, but I prescribed them anyway (off-labeling), and over the past few years there have been a few medications which have been given an FDA approval for fibromyalgia. I will be talking about the progression of my understanding of fibromyalgia and how my medication prescribing practices have changed as you read further into the book.

What is our next medication that is added to our anchor (tricyclic antidepressant) medication? This is where the road branches. The true answer to this question is we then have to recognize the hierarchy of residual symptoms and tailor our next choice of drug to the prevailing symptom or symptoms. There are so many potential scenarios of residual, persistent, or partially treated symptoms that exist, even after the sleep process has been partially or completely improved. For the sake of moving forward and connecting with the reader, who has most likely been experiencing this problem for years, let us say residual symptoms include chronic fatigue, headaches, anxiety, depression, continued joint and muscle pain, night-time muscle cramp and restless leg syndrome. These are features which fibromyalgia patients frequently experience; this is not an exaggeration of clinical features. I encounter these issues with my patients on a daily basis.

Keep in mind, when patients come to me, they often do not volunteer these symptoms, and they may just tell me about a few of them. When I initially sit down with a patient, it really only takes me a few questions to figure out the direction of the office visit. I tend to ask all the appropriate questions and they are usually just saying "yes" to all the questions. This is important not only for me, but also for the patient, because in a very short period of time, they get the impression that finally there is a doctor who understands where they are coming from, and they get the sense that something positive is about to happen. I like to think of it as a long, unsuccessful journey coming to an end, or the beginning of a new journey, but this time they have a tour guide who knows the region. I tell patients up-front, this is a journey that I am willing to take with them; but it will be a journey. Things are not going to turn around overnight or even in weeks. However, I do tell them, I will not give up; I will do my part to help them. They do, however, have to do their part, too. They have to be a good patient.

What is "my" definition of a good patient? In my book, a good patient is one that is cooperative, friendly, asks appropriate questions, takes their medications, as prescribed, keeps appointments, does their blood work and other studies as directed, and yes, I will say it, because it is the truth, pays their bills in a reasonable time period; and, if unable, at least notifies the office, so that special arrangements can be made.

Getting back to our patient example, with the persistent multitude of symptoms; where do we go from here? My approach is to look at each individual symptom and look for where the next added medication can potentially address more than one of the symptoms. I want to take advantage of the multiple potential benefits an individual medication may possess. With this in mind, I am often thinking about off-label use of a medication. I know that there will not be any specific medication out there (labeled or off-labeled) that is going to address all symptoms, but experience has showed me you can get a lot of mileage from even one well positioned medication.

When prescribing medication, I always try to take my patient's finances into consideration. It is not uncommon for many of my patients to be on several medications I have prescribed, as well as, a host of other medications from one or more other physicians. Even $10.00 co-pays add up. Couple this to the fixed incomes and I feel a personal responsibility to be cognizant of these issues towards my patients. Upfront, I tell the patient, I try to use generic medications whenever possible. I also tell them about non-generic alternatives just so they get the full story. Every now and then I get a patient that tells me, "I can't take generic medications." If that is the case, I am not going to argue with them, they will get the brand name. I preach what I practice and I practice what I preach.

For the medications, I prescribe for fibromyalgia and chronic pain, generics are fine. Keep in mind there are medications, out there I prescribe, where there are no generics. In this situation, I try to give samples when possible. With many of the non-generic medications, the pharmaceutical representatives will bring discount coupons to the office that can be given to the patients. Given the example of a patient experiencing the triad of muscle pain, muscle spasm and restless legs, my choice of medication to address all of the symptoms would be a muscle relaxant. Which one? Well, it does not really matter, I have prescribed them all. My specific choice of medication will be based on prior drug experience; did the patient ever use the drug in the past, for what reason, and what was the response? Drug formularies, a list of medications which are covered by the insurance plan, will indicate which medications will be affordable regarding co-pays for the patient with medical insurance.

The frequency of taking the medication will depend on the symptoms; dosing of muscle relaxants may vary from one to four times a day, depending on the specific medication. I never prescribe a dose more frequent or higher than outlined in the package insert, I might, however, lower the frequency of the medication, depending on the clinical features. An example of this would be if, a patient has muscle cramps at night, as well as, restless legs which interfere with sleep. In this situation, I may prescribe a muscle relaxant which is conventionally dosed 3-4 times a day, but for only one tablet to be taken at bedtime.

Remember, I am talking about a clinical process and concept. The concept that in this situation (in my experience), a muscle relaxant is indicated; it does not matter which muscle relaxant is used, as long as one is used. Whether it is effective or not is another story; success may depend on a dose adjustment or possibly a change to a different muscle relaxant. I have to see how the patient responds and where the dust settles. In many of my patients, in this situation, the muscle relaxant treats both processes; nocturnal muscle spasms and the restless leg syndrome. Another important benefit, many of these patients derive from the muscle relaxant, is it often helps with the sleep process. This may be related to the impact these medications have on the sleep pattern (I sometimes use these medications as first-line therapy), or the patients may just sleep better because the restless legs and nocturnal muscle spasms are effectively treated and they are not being awakened by these issues.

In any event, if the medication is well tolerated and the patient improves, I am pleased with the results, as is the patient. The most common side effect, and it is not often, from taking the muscle relaxant before going to bed, is that the patient may feel a bit drowsy in the morning. Sometimes, this phenomenon resolves after a few doses; after the body has gotten used to the medication. If this problem persists, I tell the patient to just take the medication 1-2 hours earlier, this usually does the trick. If the side effect persists, I will need to change muscle relaxants. I always will warn the patient this may occur, so they know what to expect and what to do if this situation develops. Just because this side effect may occur with one muscle relaxant, does not mean a change of muscle relaxant will cause the same side effect. I tell the patient the potential exists, but in most situations a medication switch is well tolerated. This may not always be the case and a few different muscle relaxants may need to be tried. If, multiple muscle relaxants cause the same side effect(s), I may need to switch to an entirely different class of medication. Sometimes one medication may not handle the problem, and additional medications may need to be added to the drug regimen.

Keeping in mind, we are dealing with our example patient who was started on the tricyclic antidepressant (amitriptyline) to address the abnormal sleep pattern. I had prescribed, at a subsequent visit, a muscle relaxant (taken at bed time), to address residual symptoms of nocturnal muscle cramps, restless legs, and also to assist the amitriptyline with the sleep process. In this specific case example, the patient now reports they are sleeping even better; and they are waking up more refreshed. I specifically ask about the sleep process at the beginning of the visit; this will be my starting point because all of the other features of fibromyalgia will be directly affected by the quality of the sleep process.

This also holds true for patients with chronic pain syndromes, whether we are dealing with chronic back pain, pain from peripheral neuropathy, peripheral joint degenerative arthritis or any process associated with ongoing chronic pain, since chronic painful conditions often disturb the sleep process. Keep in mind, pain from a chronic condition does not go away when it is time to go to sleep. Anything which interferes with the sleep cycle will cause the same features of fibromyalgia; in this situation the diagnostic term used is "secondary fibromyalgia" in which another condition is the cause of the fibromyalgia symptoms. When addressing either primary fibromyalgia or secondary fibromyalgia basic principles of treatment hold true. Not only, does the sleep process need to be addressed, but also in these situations, it is the primary painful condition that also must be addressed too.

As an example, a person who has chronic back pain, with or without a history of back surgery (back surgeries are often not successful) usually sleeps very poorly. They wake up exhausted; why would they not, since they were unable to experience a refreshed restorative sleep process; just like the patient with "primary" fibromyalgia. Now, as a result of not sleeping well, this person with chronic back pain, in addition to the chronic back pain issue, also develops features of fibromyalgia. However, aside from the similarities between these two types of patients, there are differences in the way that the medication regimen should be approached. Still, keeping with our example of our patient who suffers from lower back pain, the initial approach needs to focus on the lower back pain process. The etiology of the back pain needs to be identified. How long has the problem been present? Chronic back pain is probably there to stay; something needs to be done to alleviate the discomfort.

For the sake of keeping focused on chronic pain issues, I will skip the varieties of acute back pain, which thankfully, resolves in most people. Is the back pain due to a trauma? Is there litigation involved? These cases, in particular, tend to be messy because lawyers are involved, and it always is difficult to treat these patients because it often is hard to tell what is real or not, especially, if there are a multitude of symptoms, yet a paucity of clinical, laboratory and physical findings. Whether there is something truly there or not, it does not help their legal case, if my treatment plan is getting them better. Please do not get me wrong; people really do sustain serious and permanent injuries from all types of trauma; not only from motor vehicle accidents, but from such situations as on-the-job industrial accidents, or slipping in a public setting, such as, a shop or restaurant.

I also am quite aware of the fact, a person could injure their back and every imaging study, including: plain x-rays, CT scans and even MRI's can be completely normal showing no signs of injury. I see this all the time, and these patients have to be taken seriously, which I do. I often have patients referred to me with back pain that has had every possible test done to identify the source; all studies being normal. However, just because the studies are normal does not mean that the back pain does not exist. I usually feel quite bad for these patients because in many situations, the problem has been going on for years and nobody wants to treat it "effectively" because the various imaging studies are not correlating with the patient's symptoms. Sometimes, these patients have been suffering for years and they have never even had one imaging study! Unfortunately, the fact of the matter is the spine is quite a complex structure. With trauma and degenerative spine conditions, all it takes is a microscopic portion of a spinal nerve to be irritated and this can be associated with ongoing debilitating pain, whereby, the pathologic process is not big enough to be identified by any of the presently available imaging studies.

In any event, with our example of chronic back pain, the pain needs to be addressed. In many situations, once the back pain is brought to more tolerable levels, the fibromyalgia symptoms usually significantly improve or resolve.

Let us talk about specific medications, labeled and off-labeled, available for sleep. Early on, in the beginning of my educational process as a Rheumatologist, which continues with each passing day, I heavily relied on the use of tricyclic antidepressants to aid in the sleep process. I still use these medications in a variety of my patients for different reasons. Some of these medications have been used by my patients for years and they continue to derive ongoing benefits. One of the nice features, of this class of medication, is they can be quite effective for sleep; an off-labeled indication. They are usually well tolerated, are generic (low cost) and have a good safety profile. Of course, there are reasons why some patients should not take this class of medication, but this will be determined by the healthcare provider.

When reading the package insert or information sheet (which comes with the medication from the pharmacy), do not get caught up in the warnings. If you read about all the potential side effects, you will not want to take the medication. Just take the medication as prescribed by the healthcare provider. I always tell my patients to just take the medication, as directed, and if a problem develops, to stop taking it and contact me; we will discuss the problem and determine if it is related to the medication or something else.

Do not expect your doctor to be handing out samples of these medications; this class of medication will not be sampled by a drug rep to the physician's office. I always like to give out samples when the opportunity is there. Remember this concept: I possibly could give out samples of a non-generic medication, but the problem is, I will not be able to furnish the medication to patients on a regular basis. Non-generic medications (brand names) are not cheap. If the free sample brand name medication is helpful, the patient will subsequently need to purchase refills of this expensive medication; this will certainly be an issue for most of my patients. This is why I prefer to prescribe generic medications to my patients. In the short and long-run, this will be better for the patient. There is nothing more frustrating than giving a patient a medication sample, having it work well, and then the patient cannot afford the expensive co-pay; it is like taking candy away from a child!

Aside from amitriptyline, there are other medications, which fall into the family of tricyclic antidepressants, such as, doxepin, desipramine and nortriptyline. When I prescribe each of these medications, I use the start low and go slow concept, usually beginning with each of these medications at a starting dose of 10mg-25mg, to be taken just before going to sleep. I will titrate the dose at weekly intervals by 25mg increments; usually not going higher than 200mg at night. Keep in mind that the ultimate dose will depend on several variables such as effectiveness at a specific dose, side effects and other medications the patient is presently taking. Common side effects of these medications include: morning drowsiness (which usually improves with continued usage or taking the medication one to two hours earlier in the evening), dry mouth and constipation. There are a host of other potential side effects which can occur, but these represent the most common. The other thing, to keep in mind, is most people do not have any adverse side effects with these medications.

I really do not have any specific preference regarding the use of one tricyclic antidepressant over another. Having had an adverse reaction to one of these medications does not mean the same reaction will occur with one of the other medications. I often will move along to one of the other medications, if my initial choice is either not effective or poorly tolerated. There are certainly situations where specific adverse reactions will steer me "away" from the entire class of the medication. For example, if a patient had an anaphylactic (life threatening allergic reaction) to amitriptyline, I would not prescribe one of the other tricyclic medications, as previously mentioned, as a substitute. This is a situation where I would not take the chance of having a similar adverse reaction, as this could create a life threatening situation.

Tricyclic antidepressants can sometimes be associated with a cardiac arrhythmia (abnormal heart rhythm); some abnormal rhythms can be life threatening. If this situation developed with the use of one of these medications, I would not use one of the others for the obvious reason. Also, if I have a patient with a known history of cardiac arrhythmia I would completely avoid this class of medication. This is why it is very important for me to take a good history, during the initial evaluation; it is also important for me to know about new medical events since the last visit. Patients often will forget to mention significant past medical events. It is important for the physician to get this information from the patient during the office visit. By taking a good medication review, I can get a good sense of what other medical conditions are being treated just by knowing about the medications that are being taken. Because certain medications are prescribed in an off-labeled fashion, I often will ask the patient specifically why they are taking that particular medication.

These days, I am less likely to address poor sleep with the "initial" use of a tricyclic antidepressant, only because there are newer medications that are specifically designed for "sleep." Do not get me wrong; I still have many patients who are on tricyclic antidepressants for sleep, but as the years have passed and new medications have come onto the market, some now in generic form, my preferences have changed. One reason why I like to start out with more conventional sleep aids, that is, ones that have a specific FDA indication for sleep, is because some patients are resistant to the concept that I will be prescribing them an "antidepressant"; this class of medication is not acceptable to some patients. Before I mention that I want to prescribe an antidepressant for sleep, I give my sermon about the sleep cycle abnormality that occurs in fibromyalgia and chronic pain patients, and how this needs to be corrected for the healing process to begin. I then talk about how medications are used in an off-labeled manner, and then, I ease into the concept that to achieve proper sleep I will need to prescribe an antidepressant. I then state how these medications have been quite effective, in the thousands of patients, whom I have prescribed them to over the past twenty or so years, their safety profile and their low cost. By this time most, people are on board and we can begin the journey.

SECTION TWO

Sleep Aids

Over the past several years, one of my favorite sleeping aids, to pre-scribe for my patients, has been zolpidem (Ambien). This is a medica-tion that has been on the market for many years; it specifically does have an FDA indication for sleep. I have found this medication to be quite helpful for many of my patients. I actually prefer this medication as an initial starting point over the tricyclic antidepressants for several reasons. First, it works well. People do not get hung up with this medi-cation, as they sometimes do, when I tell them I want to prescribe an antidepressant. Second, patients are less likely to get the two most com-mon side effects with Ambien, as compared to the tricyclic antidepres-sants; dry mouth and morning drowsiness. Third, what I have found with the use of Ambien, over the tricyclic antidepressants, is people have an easier time waking up in the middle of the night and getting right back to sleep when compared to those on the tricyclic medications; this is important, especially if the person taking the Ambien has small chil-dren at home, or a person has to get up frequently to urinate at night, as in the case of elderly men who have prostate issues. Keep in mind, this is not a set rule and each person will respond to each medication dif-ferently; this is just a non-scientific observation I have made throughout the years. Personal experience, with regard to managing my patients, is a major factor which determines how I practice medicine.

Whenever a "new" medication reaches the general public, whether it will be effective in a particular patient or not, one thing is certain, it will not be cheap! Drug companies can easily invest hundreds of mil-lions of dollars into the research and development of a new product; they intend to get their money back, and then some. This is why there is no such thing as an inexpensive brand name drug, which means, there are no available equivalent generic medications to this specific product at this specific time. The law states, when a pharmaceutical company has a patent on a new medication, there is a long period of time during which no other pharmaceutical company can copy that drug. This protected time period, a period of about 15-20 years, gives the pharmaceutical company noncompetitive time to recoup their investment and hopefully (for them) to make a killing, I know, bad word choice! [Note: By the time the drug reaches the market there will usually be 11-13 years left on the patent.]

Now, a few short comments about generic versus the non-generic (brand name) counterpart. The argument that will be stated regarding brand versus generic is the fact that generics may not have the same "bioavailability" compared to the brand name medication. The term "bioavailability" means the amount of medication the body truly absorbs given a particular dose of medication. For example, we can state, when dealing with a brand name drug, the amount of medication that is available to work on the body after absorption is 100%; for the amount that should be absorbed. Once in the body this medication then has to do its magic. On the other hand, with regard to the generic counterpart medication, once it gets absorbed, given the same dose of medication, it may not have the same effect on the body as the brand name counterpart. The same dose of the generic may, for example, be only 80% as effective as the brand name medication.

There are allowances with drug absorption (bioavailability), that the FDA accepts regarding variations of a given product between different pharmaceutical companies making the same generic medication. Some generic medications are made by different companies, and the bioavailability of each medication may, certainly vary from one company to another. I have had patients tell me, certain generics are not effective when they switch from one pharmaceutical company to the other; this is a phenomenon that occurs at the level of the drug store. The medication contracts between the pharmacies and the pharmaceutical companies can change from year-to-year; hence, the manufacturer change from one generic brand to another. Sometimes, in this situation, the patient may need to obtain prescriptions from multiple pharmacies just to stay with their "brand" of "generic." The one thing, I can tell you about sleep aids, is it will become evident very quickly (a few doses), whether a change from brand to generic or generic to a different generic will be effective or detrimental.

One simple example, of the variation between generic products, is in the case of the Duragesic (fentanyl) narcotic pain patch. The Mylan brand generic patch (at this point in time) has a better adhesive than the other available generic brand (Watson); this is what my patients tell me. If the patch does not adhere to the body properly, the medication will not work effectively because the delivery of this medication is transdermal (absorbed through the skin). If, the patch does not stick properly, this will reduce the bioavailability(less absorption), and the medication will not work. The brand name (Duragesic) has no adherence problems, but is very expensive. In this situation, when I prescribe this patch, I specifically write on the prescription "Mylan brand only," a special request for a particular generic medication; the generic cost will be no different to the patient. These patients may have to go to a different pharmacy to get this medication, depending upon whether this generic brand is carried by their regular pharmacy.

I do, however, need to make the following statement: in my practice, with regard to dealing with fibromyalgia and other chronic painful conditions, the concept of generic versus non-generic is not really an issue (in my opinion) for the management of pain in my patients. Even, if there is a real issue of bioavailability between generic versus non-generics, I easily can adjust the doses of specific medications to compensate for any potential (or perceived) differences when I change a medication from brand to generic. There are situations, where I hear from my colleagues (cardiologist, endocrinologist and neurologist) where they believe certain generic medications should not be substituted over brand name medications for certain conditions they treat. Here is a situation where quality and bioavailability of a generic over a brand medication could have serious implications. If a neurologist were to tell me, the brand name medication controls seizures better than the generic; I would do what it takes to obtain the brand name medication. There is a big difference between a poor night of sleep and a seizure. There is no such thing as a convenient seizure. The same concept goes for the field of cardiology. There are certain cardiac arrhythmias (abnormal heart rhythm) that can be lethal. In this situation, I would want to take the medication which the cardiologist feels works the best and they may advise a brand over a generic in this situation. I also have heard from the endocrinologist, it is their opinion, certain brands of thyroid medication work better than generics. In these situations the patient has to trust and put their faith in what the doctor tells them.

Getting back to Ambien, there is a generic form of this medication. Ambien comes in two forms, an immediate release and a sustained release. The immediate release has a generic form (zolpidem). This medication comes in two strengths, 5 mg and 10 mg tablets. I have not had any patients notice any difference between the immediate release form of generic versus non-generic Ambien. Most patients will need to take the higher dose (10 mg tablet). Some may get by with the 5 mg tablet. The benefit, for the patient that only needs the 5 mg tablet to accomplish the job of a good night's sleep, is that I can prescribe a 10 mg tablet and they can cut it in half; it is a little extra work, but in this situation, 30 tablets will actually last for two months, a savings to the patient, which is always welcomed.

There is another form of Ambien called Ambien CR which since the publication of the first edition of this book has become available as a generic. This medication comes in two doses, 6.25 mg and 12.5 mg. These tablets should not be cut. This tablet is designed differently than Ambien (immediate release) whereby the tablet contains two layers of the active ingredient; the outer layer is designed to break away quickly from the tablet so the body quickly absorbs a higher dose of the medication to get the patient more rapidly to sleep. The inner layer is absorbed slowly to keep the patient asleep during the rest of the night. So, you are probably wondering, is there a difference between the effectiveness of Ambien CR over the Ambien immediate release? Here is my non-biased observation, some patients tell me they feel the Ambien CR works better than the immediate release, for others, they feel no difference.

[Note: Since the first publication of this book the FDA has issued a warning stating that women using the 10mg dose of Ambien (zolpidem) are at increased risk of being involved in motor vehicle accidents (while driving) the next morning. My observation throughout the years is that the vast majority of all of my patients(male and female) taking Ambien need to be on the 10mg dose for it to be effective, as opposed to the 5mg dose which is recommended by the FDA for females. I always ask all of my patients on Ambien, and document in the medical record with each office visit, if they are having any issues with morning driving if they are taking Ambien the previous evening.]

Another medication that is specifically designed (FDA approved) for sleep is Lunesta. This is a medication that has been on the market for several years. This medication does not have a generic form (at this time), so it will not be inexpensive; the price will depend upon your insurance co-pay; providing you have medical insurance. This medication comes in three doses, 1 mg, 2 mg and 3 mg tablets. The tablet is to be taken just as the person is going to bed, the same as for Ambien and other sleep aids. One common side effect, of this medication, is it can cause the patient to experience a sour taste in the mouth, usually experienced in the morning. This phenomenon will sometimes subside with continued use. It can be counteracted by having the patient take a mint or citrus candy, in the morning, when they wake up. You might think it is inconvenient to have to take measures to counteract this side effect, but keep in mind, if this medication happens to be a home run for the patient with regard to adequately addressing a poor sleep process, it will be a small price to pay. It is unusual for patients to stop taking this medication because of the sour taste side effect. In my practice, Lunesta is certainly not the first sleep aid I reach for, only because it is not generic, and I can usually accomplish correcting an abnormal sleep process with another (or other) generic medications. When I put a patient on Lunesta, it is because I am running out of options and the patient is aware that this medication will be costing more than the previous medications I have already prescribed for sleep. Do not get me wrong, I have nothing against Lunesta, I think it is a good medication; I have many patients who successfully use this medication. I just try to be cost conscious, while managing my patient's medical conditions, whenever possible. One little trick I will use with Lunesta is to prescribe a 2 mg or 3 mg tablet with the intention of having the patient take only half of the tablet, or use the full tablet if the half tablet is not effective. For example, I will prescribe a 2 mg tablet and have the patient start off with half of the tablet (1 mg). If this is effective, the prescription will last the patient two months. In this situation what would be considered too much money to spend for a month supply of a medication becomes more reasonable and affordable if it turns into a two month supply for the same co-pay as a one month supply. Cutting the tablet will increase the potential for the patient to experience the sour taste in the mouth; that is what some patients tell me. I simply caution my patients about this possibility.

One last FDA approved insomnia medication, which I prescribe, is a drug called Rozerem; generically called ramelteon. [Note: There is no generic form for this medication at this time.] This medication works by a different mechanism for helping the sleep cycle as compared to the other drugs, which already have been mentioned. Rozerem binds to the melatonin receptors in the brain. It is believed that stimulating these receptors helps a person get into a deep sleep. Melatonin can also be purchased over-the-counter, but the effect of Rozerem will be several folds more potent than any type of melatonin that can be obtained over-the-counter. This medication comes as an 8 mg tablet, which is taken at bedtime. Unfortunately, my experience, with this medication, is that it has not been very effective for sleep for the vast majority of my patients who have taken this medication. However, where I have seen the value, of Rozerem, is when I prescribe this medication in combination with another sleep aid (any of the other aids); in this situation it has helped many of my patients with insomnia. It is like the icing on the cake; like adding hamburger helper to ground beef. The problem, in this situation, is this medication is not inexpensive; taking two non-generic sleep aids concomitantly can cost a fair amount of money. The drug company does have discount coupons which the doctor's office should have; coupons often bring the cost down to what you would pay for a generic medication. Also, many pharmaceutical companies offer discount coupons that can be obtained through their company website.

SECTION THREE

Muscle Relaxants

Muscle relaxants often are helpful for sleep disorders, either as a primary sleep medication or in combination with other sleep medications. Simply put, muscle relaxants cause the muscles to relax. A muscle which is not relaxed is tense; it may also be in spasm. Either of these two processes is uncomfortable. Aside from experiencing pain during the day from this process, it often will continue into and throughout the night, not only causing pain, but inability to sleep.

Patients often tell me, they hurt more at night; why is this? I do have my own theory about this and this is what I tell people: during the day, we are active, doing things, going places, and just taking care of everything we have to do for ourselves and others. The body can only process so much information at one time; the same goes for pain sensation. If you are concentrating on driving a car, grocery shopping, conversing with the barber or hair stylist, this is a form of distraction from pain. I am not saying that these activities take pain away; they are distractions of pain. Aside from your chronic painful condition, which is still there, the process of focusing on something else, whatever that may be, forces you to not be so focused on your baseline discomfort. Now, at the end of the day, and you are unwinding from a busy (or not so busy day), you begin to focus more on yourself; you are more in tune to the constant pains you experience on a day-to-day basis. The distractions of the day are over.

Also, in a negative fashion, this time of the day gives certain people an opportunity to worry about various issues, which in turn, can exacerbate stress which does have a physiologic effect on the body; not a good one. This process can actually exacerbate baseline discomfort creating a time of the day, which is characterized by more pain, which certainly is not helpful when the immediate focus is on sleep. Stress often causes or exacerbates muscle spasm, which causes discomfort. In my opinion, there are certain situations where a muscle relaxant is the most appropriate sleep aid. Once again, I find it a key issue to determine what causes the sleep disturbance; is it chronic pain, anxiety, stress, depression, sleep apnea or just primary insomnia. The choice of medication(s) prescribed will be determined on the basis of a good medical history and physical examination, not on the basis of a person saying they cannot sleep. Believe it or not, most patients, who sleep poorly, do not even mention the fact they cannot sleep properly; I am the one who usually asks the questions about sleep and sleep quality.

There are plenty of muscle relaxants available; most are actually generic. The appropriate dosing of muscle relaxants can vary from patient to patient. When looking at dispensing instructions from the PDR (Physician's Desk Reference), most muscle relaxants are prescribed three to four times a day when treating muscle spasms. However, I often will prescribe these medications for just nighttime dosing, when my main intention is to use them in an off-labeled fashion, as either a primary or adjunctive (in addition to) medication for sleep disturbance.

Looking to the generically available category of medications, I prescribe for sleep, brings me to an old favorite, Klonopin (brand name), generically known as clonazepam. This is a medication that is not specifically FDA approved for insomnia, as is Ambien and Lunesta. However, I have been prescribing this medication for years to patients, who experience poor sleep and a host of other related and non-related conditions. This is one of those medications where I try to hit more than one bird with one stone.

Clonazepam is a medication that falls under the family of a benzo-diazepine, the same class as valium. I assume that it is for this reason many doctors do not like to prescribe this medication; when they do they dole it out in small quantities. In the long run, when inadequate amounts of sleep aids are prescribed, this type of medication pre-scribing will be ineffective and potentially frustrating to both patient and physician: frustrating to the physician because they will not want to prescribe it on a regular ongoing basis; frustrating to the patient because they will need it every night. Then, the patient will have to ration their medication allotment and the sleep pattern and process will be inconsistent. If the doctor only gives the patient 15 tablets per month, I can assure you, the patient potentially will experience only 15 nights of quality sleep that month. Sleep aids only work the night they are taken. You cannot get two days of mileage from one dose. You have to pay the toll to get onto the sleep highway each night!

When I prescribe clonazepam for sleep, I am doing it in an off-labeled fashion. Other benefits of this medication are: it is often quite effective for the management of other conditions, such as, muscle spasms, restless legs, muscle cramps, stress and anxiety. If I have a patient, who has fibromyalgia or chronic pain, who also suffers from restless legs, stress and/or anxiety, clonazepam is a good choice of drug to use in this patient. I can assure you, I will be prescribing this medication in a way that a dose will be able to be taken every night (the dosage strength will vary from patient to patient). Sometimes I will prescribe this medication in a pattern by which the patient may be taking it two to three times a day; for the patient who needs this medication for reasons other than sleep, such as, stress, anxiety, or muscle spasms.

When prescribing this medication, I usually start with 0.5 mg to be taken just as the patient attempts to get into bed. I will instruct the patient to upwardly adjust the medication by increments of 0.5 mg doses on a weekly basis, noting I will be seeing the patient for a two week follow-up appointment. Subsequent dosing adjustments will depend on the patient's progress on the medication. I tell the patient to stop the medication and call me if a problem develops while taking the new medication; we can discuss over the phone what is going on, and I can, at that time, usually determine if the problem is related to the new drug or something else.

Another oldie, but goodie medication, which I often prescribe for sleep, is Halcion (triazolam). This is a medication that has been around for decades. It falls under the family of a benzodiazepine. I have been prescribing this medication to many of my patients for years, either by itself or in combination with other sleep aids. I think one of the problems, physicians have, is in writing sleep aids for continuous use. The vast majority of patients, who have sleeping problems, will need to take "something" for sleep on a regular basis. Patients will often tell me their healthcare provider will only prescribe 10-15 sleeping aid tablets per month. I certainly do not understand this thinking on the part of the practitioner; actually I do. There is one of two things going on here: either the healthcare provider does not understand the concept that people with sleep disorders need to take something "each night" for sleep; or the healthcare provider feels uncomfortable about prescribing the medication the way it really needs to be prescribed (or both). Either way, the patient suffers.

The fact of the matter is, many healthcare providers are afraid to write for certain medications on a regular basis. These medications are usually opioids (narcotics), benzodiazepines (Klonopin, Valium and Halcion) and sleep specific medications, such as, Ambien and Lunesta. Whenever there are warnings about these medications leading to "addiction" and "dependence," this scares doctors. Unfortunately, we live in a litigious society; it does not help when every other commercial on TV is about suing a drug company. Quite simply put, doctors are afraid of being sued. They have concerns; they will be accused of creating a drug addict. Most doctors feel uncomfortable in this arena of medication prescribing. It is an interesting phenomenon, how a doctor can be practicing for 20-30 years and yet have deficiencies in what would be considered a basic aspect of medicine. When you think about it, how can one become skilled at treating "complex" sleeping issues when they cannot even address, what I would consider "simple" sleep issues in a fair number of patients? I am not doctor bashing here; I just am pointing out a reality. I do not claim to be all knowing in the field of medicine, far from it. I have had the luxury throughout the years to practice within a specific aspect of medicine; there are, however, a lot of medical problems I do not treat in my practice, hence the need for a primary care provider.

The types of patients, who are sent to me, go beyond the experience of the PCP (primary care physician). As a specialist in Rheumatology, I did two extra years of medical training at Dartmouth as a Rheumatology Fellow; specifically learning about and how to treat connective tissue disorders. Obviously, one can learn only so much in two years. My Rheumatology Fellowship training at Dartmouth gave me the tools to think like a Rheumatologist and prepare me for a career in the management of connective tissue diseases. The real learning, however, began after my formal training; a journey which has covered over two decades of private practice and continues with each passing day. I always feel I learn something from my patients on a daily basis. I constantly have to be thinking and managing patients outside-of-the-box.

Getting back to Halcion (triazolam), the starting dose of this medication is 0.125 mg to be taken at bedtime. Sometimes, I need to increase the dose to 0.25 mg. I sometimes will have to combine this with another sleep aid that is already on board, or this may be the first sleep aid I prescribe to the patient. Once again, keep in mind, this is a medication many healthcare providers will not be prescribing because of reasons already discussed. You can see why addressing sleep issues, with patients, is so difficult for the patient; the person writing (or not writing) the prescription is half the problem.

When I was in Fellowship, I often prescribed Flexoril (generically known as cyclobenzaprine), for the sleep disturbance of fibromyalgia. I still prescribe and have many patients who take this medication. I usually prescribe this medication as a 10 mg dose to be taken at bedtime. Sometimes the dose has to be downwardly adjusted to 5 mg at bedtime, if excessive drowsiness develops in the morning. Also, in an elderly patient or a patient who tells me that they are sensitive to medications, I will start off on the 5 mg dose, giving the patient instructions to increase the dose to 10 mg in a few days, if the dose is tolerated but there has not been any significant improvement. Also, I may start the patient on the 5 mg dose depending upon what other medications are on board, since the addition of one more drug, which acts on the central nervous system, may go a long way on the lower dose. I always can increase the dose, if needed. The last thing any of my elderly patients need is for me to give them a medication that causes them to get dizzy, fall and break a hip. In the elderly population, when it comes to medication prescribing, I prefer to use the rule of start low and go slow. I am forever explaining this concept to my patients. People often get frustrated when they take a medication and do not get an immediate response.

There is actually a 5 mg Flexoril tablet that is generic. When I want a patient to start on the 5mg of Flexoril, I just tell them to cut the generic 10 mg tablet in half. If things work out on the 5 mg tablet, they will have a two month supply for the generic price of a one month script. The virtues of this type of prescription writing have already been described; the benefits are self-evident. There is an extended release, non-generic form of Flexoril called Amrix. This is a 15 mg tablet designed for once-a-day dosing. When I prescribe Flexoril (cyclobenzaprine) for a once-a-day, bedtime dose, I prefer it to be the immediate release form; I am not looking for 24 hour muscle relaxation, just a sleep aid. Of course, when the sleep is accomplished, the patients usually feel better; there is less muscle discomfort. Remember, non-generic medications are not cheap and part of my mission, as a physician, is to effectively treat my patients in a cost effective manner. It can be done and I have been doing it successfully for years!

The fact of the matter is I really do not have any specific preference when it comes to prescribing a muscle relaxant for my patients. Once again, my decision making process for prescribing all medications is based on prior medication usage, contraindications, other medications that are on board, and of course affordability. Names of some commonly prescribed muscle relaxants in my practice include: Soma (carisprodal), Baclofen (lioresal), Valium (diazepam) and Klonopin (clonazepam) to name just a few. All of these medications are available in generic form. Once again, these classes of medications are the type that many healthcare providers would feel uncomfortable writing on a regular basis. When you compound this issue with the fact the medication is being prescribed in an off-labeled manner, this creates an unfavorable situation for the patient. Any time a medication interferes with the prescribing pattern or comfort level of the healthcare provider this is not going to be working in favor of the patient.

Muscle relaxants are quite helpful not only for sleep; I often prescribe them for my patients with restless leg syndrome. In this condition the sleep process is interrupted by nocturnal (nighttime) jerking of the legs. This can adversely affect the sleep pattern and cause significant discomfort in the legs, causing the patient to get up and out of bed for prolonged periods of time until it settles down; this is not a good thing to be happening throughout the night. Restless leg syndrome, in and of itself, is enough to be responsible for insomnia in some patients.

For the treatment of restless leg syndrome, there are a few drugs on the market, which are specifically FDA approved for the management of this condition. All of these medications are effective for most people. Discount cards are sometimes available at the prescriber's office, providing the pharmaceutical rep has given them to the doctor; they usually do, because it is in their best interest for the doctor to prescribe their medications, since their job (sales of their product) and bonuses depend on it. Unfortunately, sometimes the drug reps make the discount cards available to the physician, but the physician fails to give them to the patient. My advice to the reader is, if you are given a new prescription; ask the healthcare provider if the medication has a generic form. If a generic is not available, ask if there is another medication that can be used as an alternative. Ask if they have any medication coupons or discount cards. Sometimes doctors write prescriptions without thinking about the cost of the medication.

Another issue, with regard to prescription writing, is the same medication may cost different amounts depending on the specific insurance company's medication benefits. I try to keep track of the various costs of medications, which I prescribe to my patients. Even when I am prescribing generics, which by now you can see I do as often as possible without compromising patient care; I ask my patients what the prescription cost. I do not want my patients to have sticker shock at the pharmacy. Not only is this stressful to patients, but also embarrassing, when they have to say to the pharmacist they cannot afford the medication.

From the physician's side of this story, this is only going to generate a phone call from the patient explaining the financial predicament, which will then lead the physician to review the chart; engage in a dialogue (which could last a while), require a note to be charted;

and then a prescription will either have to be called into the pharmacy or a script sent by mail to the patient. In the end, everyone will be going through a hassle, which could have been avoided, if the initial prescription written was well thought out. As a busy physician, I can tell you, I strive to get it all right during the patient visit.

If you ever wondered why doctors are always running late, it is usually because of all the unexpected interruptions which occur during the day. Calls come from other doctors, especially if you are a specialist like myself, patient and their family member phone calls, phone calls from pharmacies, hospitals and even solicitors, who have been able to get past my first line of defense, my receptionist. Also, sometimes (actually quite often) a follow-up appointment or even a new patient evaluation can take longer than expected. If, I have to do a procedure such as inject a joint, or a carpel tunnel injection, this adds to the time of the visit. Also, do not forget about the time needed to see pharmaceutical reps; these people are important to meet with. Of course, they want as much time as they can get to promote their product. After all, they are providing the doctor's office with free samples (of course, not generics) and discount coupons. They also provide information about their products which is geared both specifically to patients and physicians. Just about all pharmaceutical companies have programs that will provide free medications to certain patients, if medical necessity exists where limited patient income can be documented.

Restless leg syndrome is a common cause of sleep disturbance. There are two specific generic medications on the market that are specifically used for the management of restless leg syndrome. One is Requip, generically called ropinirole hydrochloride, a medication whose first FDA indication was for the treatment of Parkinson's disease, a neurologic disorder that effects movement and speech. This medication is classified as a dopamine agonist. The prescribing regimen, for this medication, varies depending on which condition is being treated. For restless legs it is dosed at night (bedtime). The starting dose is usually 0.25-0.5 mg. The dose may need to be titrated upwards depending on the patient's response to the initial dose.

I have several patients who are on this medication and they are having a good response for the management of their restless leg syndrome. The only issue, I have with this medication, is it will not have the same multiple benefits a bedtime muscle relaxant will offer the patient. It certainly may help the restless leg component, but may do nothing for muscle spasms, a non-restorative sleep process, or anxiety.

It really is important to dissect out all the issues which keep the patient from having a good night's sleep. I see no value (off the bat) from starting a patient on a bedtime muscle relaxant for addressing muscle spasms and Requip for addressing restless legs in the same patient at the same time. Why "initially" prescribe both of these medications when the muscle relaxant, as a single agent, may do the trick to address restless legs, muscle spasms and insomnia. If the patient gets a partial response to the muscle relaxant, let us say the muscle spasm and insomnia improves, but the restless legs persists, then the addition of Requip or another similar agent may then be employed. Why start out with two medications for this scenario, with two co-pays, when one drug may be all that is necessary. Also, the more drugs on board the greater the potential for side effects and drug to drug interactions. If a patient is started on two new drugs at the same time and a side effect or allergic reaction develops you may have to stop both medications and possibly have to prescribe another medication to address the newly developed adverse reaction.

Another FDA approved medication for the management of restless leg syndrome is Mirapex (pramipexole). Like Requip, this medication is also a dopamine agonist, whose initial FDA indication was for the treatment of Parkinson's disease. The dosing regimen of this medication also differs, depending on which condition is being treated. This medication, when prescribed for the management of restless leg syndrome, is also started at a low dose, 0.125 mg - 0.25 mg at bedtime. The dose may need to be titrated upwards depending on the patient's response.

There are other medications which fall under the family of dopamine agonists which are often prescribed in an off-labeled fashion for the management of restless leg syndrome, such as, the Parkinson's medication known as Sinemet (carbidopa/methyldopa).

There is a transdermal (patch) called Neupro (rotigotine transdermal system).This is different than the other medications for the management of restless leg syndrome in that this is a once a day skin patch. The dose is started at 1mg/24 hr. with a maximum dose of 3mg/ 24 hr. There are 1, 2, and 3mg patches (for the management of restless leg syndrome). [Note: I have not used this in any of my patients as of the time of this printing; I just wanted to mention it because it is out there and it has a unique delivery system for the management of restless leg syndrome.]

As you can see, just with the medications I have already mentioned, there are plenty of generic and non-generic medications available for the management of a poor sleep pattern. It is interesting to note, we have already reviewed several classes of medications, which can be quite effective for treating insomnia. It is important to identify the factors which could contribute to insomnia and, when possible, use a medication which has the potential to address more than one ailment. Sometimes, it is necessary to combine different classes of medications to achieve maximal sleep benefit. The management of sleep disturbances will be a very subjective endeavor for the healthcare provider. There are no right or wrong answers as to which drug should be used first (or avoided), or which combination of medication will work the best.

I think whatever drug or drugs are used, there needs to be some common sense employed by the healthcare provider; they need to know what questions to ask; do not reinvent the wheel; and be sure to take a good history, making particular note of previous medications which have been used and what has and has not been effective. When a patient tells me a prior medication was ineffective, I do not let the conversation about that medication come to an end. I want to know what effect the medication had on the patient. Was there a side effect? Did the medication just not work? How long was the medication taken, and most importantly, what was the dose of the medication which was felt to be ineffective?

Patients often tell me a medication was not helpful, only to learn the person was taking a low dose or sub maximal dose. The clinical effects of many of the medications, I have already discussed, are "dose dependent" (this means the clinical response to the medication is related to the dose of the medication which is being taken). For example, Klonopin (the benzodiazepine muscle relaxant) may be very effective for insomnia at 1 mg at bedtime, but in that same person the restless leg problems, may not be controlled unless the dose of Klonopin is 2 mg at night. This is an example where one medication is being used to treat two separate conditions. Another example, still using Klonopin, is the patient may not sleep well on 2 mg at bedtime, but may do quite well with 2.5 mg at bedtime. When a patient tells me a drug was not effective and they were not taking the maximal dose of that medication, I do not consider the medication to be a failure. Obviously, if the medication caused an unacceptable side effect then there is no value of revisiting that medication in the future.

Another important concept, which should not be overlooked, is the opposite of not taking enough of the medication; taking too much. When patients tell me a particular medication was not tolerated, I want to know specifically, what was the adverse reaction? Sometimes, a healthcare provider will start a medication at a dose that is a bit too high for the patient to tolerate. Even what may be considered a low dose, may need to be downwardly adjusted, so the medication will be tolerated. If a patient tells me they are very sensitive to medications, I will often start a new medication at a very low dose; sometimes at a dose which is not considered to be therapeutic. My reasoning for this is there are two things that need to be accomplished; treating the condition and tolerance of the medication. It is very important to get the medication on board and for it to be well tolerated.

This initial process is even more important than being effective in treating the condition. I would rather go low and go slow with a medication, as the dose can always be upwardly adjusted. Sometimes, the body needs time to adjust to the introduction of a new medication. It may be necessary to start on a very low dose and then slowly (in one week intervals) increase the dose (slowly) until the desired effect is attained. For example, using Klonopin might be initiated at 0.5 mg at bedtime to treat insomnia. The next morning the patient is very drowsy and it takes a few hours for that effect to wear off. Many patients will stop taking the medication at that point. When I see them for a follow-up appointment (two weeks later), they then tell me this medication was not tolerated and they want something different. I will often get a phone call before the follow-up appointment, if side effects develop when taking a new medication. After all, I did tell the patient to call me if any problems develop with the new medication. I am okay with this type of phone call. I will want to make an adjustment over the phone. Why have the patient wait a week and a half off the medication (without treatment) until the next appointment?

Given this description of side effect (morning drowsiness), I really do not want to abandon this medication, just yet. There is still great potential for the effectiveness and good tolerance of this medication. The dose just needs to be lowered. Why change to another medication where they may experience the same side effect from a new prescription, besides, they would have to make another trip to the pharmacy, pay another co-pay, or full payment for a new prescription, if they do not have prescription coverage. When a patient just stops the medication without notifying me by phone, part of the problem which I will be facing at the follow-up appointment will be to convince that patient to stick with the medication, but just to take half the dose. This would have been the instruction, if the phone call was placed to me before the follow-up visit.

The lower dose may now be well tolerated, but not effective, in addressing the sleep disorder (at the lower dose). If the lower dose is then tolerated, after a week (an arbitrary period of time) the dose then can be increased, and perhaps the higher dose will, not only, be tolerated, but also effective in addressing the insomnia. I can think of many occasions when a patient had a side effect on what would be considered a low starting dose of a medication, developed what I would consider to be a minor side effect, which could be transient if the dose is lowered, the dose is then lowered, tolerance develops, and then the dose is increased to obtain the desired positive effect. Sometimes, the dose of the medication needs to be significantly increased to achieve the desired benefit.

It is interesting to note, for many of these patients, the final achieved dose of the medication for successful management can be several folds higher than the initial low dose, which was not well tolerated. This is a good example where it is important to not abandon a drug so quickly. If every medication was stopped because of initial (modifiable) side effects, the situation of running out of appropriate medications to treat all conditions would become a major problem.

When dealing with insomnia, I am willing to give medications a chance. Not to sound insensitive to these patients, but it is my attitude that this problem has been going on for a long time; years in many circumstances. If it takes me a few weeks, to get it right for them, I consider that acceptable. Most patients initially are concerned more about making the initial connection with the doctor and to quickly develop a trust and confidence with their healthcare provider. I think it is very important, from the initial visit, that both the healthcare provider and patient have realistic expectations. I explain to my patients, I will do my best to help them. I will listen to what they have to say; I will ask what I believe are the right questions, necessary for me to effectively manage their condition. It will be a mutual journey, and it will take time. I really do believe patients do much better and actually respond better to treatment, when I outline, what I expect to take place with the medications I prescribe; kind of like a sales pitch. Trust me, I will not be conning anyone into feeling better. I truly do have to deliver from my end of the bargain.

Just one final note, with regard to the patient who may experience excessive morning drowsiness with the initial dose of the medication, where they may be reluctant to give the medication a second chance at a lower dose (they often tell me they could not function at work the next day). I tell them to give the medication another try at half the dose (just cut the tablet in half, this will not work if it is a capsule), but try it again on the weekend (or the night before a day off) where nothing special is planned for the next day.

Another concept to be aware of, when two separate medications are employed together, for example, Ambien and any of the muscle relaxants, the initial starting dose of one or both drugs may be pre-scribed, at a lower dose, than the dose that would be used if each drug was used alone because of the synergistic (additive) effect between the two medications. As a general rule, the lower the dose of a medi-cation used; the less potential of developing a side effect from that medication. Conversely, the addition of one medication may heighten the effect of another drug; this may be a good or bad thing. Treating fibromyalgia and chronic pain conditions is like making a stew. It will not taste right unless the proper ingredients are added in the right proportions. Some vegetables cost more than others; organic (brand name) will cost more than regular grown (generic). The meat may be the most expensive ingredient, and a good grade of beef (brand name) may taste much better than chuck steak (generic). Years of clinical experience has proved to me, many of my patients do quite well on complex (and non-complex) medication regimens which are composed entirely of generic medications, and the stew taste just as good!

SECTION FOUR

Nonsteroidal Anti-Inflammatory Drugs (NSAIDs)

What about an NSAID for the management of fibromyalgia? Fibromyalgia is not an inflammatory condition, there is no inflammation associated with this condition. Keep in mind, however, people with fibromyalgia may also have an associated inflammatory condition, such as, rheumatoid arthritis or lupus. Other inflammatory conditions, such as, bursitis, tendonitis and degenerative arthritis (osteoarthritis) may also coexist.

NSAIDs have three basic qualities. First, they are anti-inflammatories (they bring down inflammation). Second, they are analgesics (pain relievers) and third, they are antipyretics (they bring down fever). If you think about it, there is no inflammation associated with fibromyalgia (strictly speaking). However, we often use NSAIDs when treating patients with fibromyalgia. Why is this? Because fibromyalgia is a painful condition and, as I have just mentioned NSAIDs also work as analgesics (pain relievers). So, there may be value to using an NSAID in a patient with fibromyalgia. An NSAID may be particularly helpful in a fibromyalgia patient especially, if there is also an associated inflammatory or degenerative process, as already discussed.

As a general rule, I would not use an NSAID as an "initial" medication for the management of fibromyalgia. The NSAID may help with some of the discomfort associated with fibromyalgia, but will do nothing to address the fundamental problem of the abnormal sleep process. I certainly may prescribe an NSAID along with a sleep aid, especially if there is a concomitant inflammatory or degenerative process. There may be a situation where the sleep process is exacerbated by a painful arthritic process, such as, bursitis or tendonitis. The sleep aid will certainly have no effect on these other processes, which also need to be addressed.

The thing, one has to keep in mind, is many different classes of medications can be used to treat pain. The healthcare provider needs to look at all the options and decide which medication(s) will be the most appropriate to prescribe. As a general rule, if there is no associated inflammatory condition, which will benefit from the use of an NSAID, I prefer to use another class or several classes of medications to address fibromyalgia and other chronic painful conditions. Although, NSAIDs can be quite helpful for various inflammatory and non-inflammatory conditions, there are certain risks associated with taking these medications on a long-term and sometimes, short-term basis.

Some of the adverse effects of NSAIDs include gastric irritation and ulcer formation, which may be associated with or without bleeding. This can present, even without warning of abdominal symptoms, as an acute life threatening bleed requiring emergency hospitalization, blood transfusion and surgery. NSAIDs can affect any portion of the gastrointestinal system. If there is any history of gastritis, ulcer, or gastrointestinal bleeding one has to be very cautious with prescribing NSAIDs. There are situations, whereby, to employ an NSAID safely, one or two gastric protector medications will need to be concomitantly prescribed. There is always the risk of bleeding from both the chronic and short-term use of NSAIDs. I always explain this to my patients, to whom I prescribe NSAIDs to on a regular basis. It is important to risk stratify (classify) patients according to whom would most likely develop adverse reactions from the chronic use of NSAIDs. As a general rule, if I have a patient, who has a history of significant adverse gastrointestinal effect with the prior use of an NSAID (bleed or bowel perforation), I will most likely avoid the use of any NSAID.

As a word of caution to any of you, reading this book, who have been in this situation in the past, I strongly recommend you not take any over-the-counter NSAIDs either. I cannot tell you how many times I see patients, who are in a situation, where they have contraindications to the use of NSAIDs. Their healthcare providers know not to prescribe any NSAIDs. The problem is these patients think it is okay to use the over-the-counter (OTC) NSAIDs, since a prescription is not needed. Some people are not aware that they are taking an NSAID. With the way that over-the-counter NSAIDs are advertised on TV, people think these are harmless pain medications, and have no idea these medications are NSAIDs. Remember, over-the-counter Advil and Motrin are ibuprofen (NSAID); and Aleve is naproxen sodium (Naprosyn), also an NSAID. These medications are readily available for public consumption without the need of a prescription.

Aside from the potential issue of varying degrees of inflammation to the gastrointestinal system, NSAIDs can adversely affect other organ systems of the body. NSAIDs can have negative effects on kidney function. If a person has renal (kidney) insufficiency to begin with, seen commonly in elderly, diabetic and hypertensive patients, NSAIDs can create or exacerbate renal insufficiency. In some situations, NSAIDs have been associated with outright renal failure. As a general rule, the renal insufficiency associated with the use of NSAIDs usually is reversible, by either discontinuing the medication or lowering the dose. Sometimes, NSAIDs may cause blood to appear in the urine. [Note: Bleeding could be either "macroscopic bleeding," being able actually to see blood in the urine; or "microscopic bleeding," where the blood is only visible under the microscope.]

The effect that NSAIDs can have on the kidneys can occur quite rapidly. I always want to know the level of renal function in any patient to whom I plan on prescribing an NSAID for a long or sometimes, short period of time. Sometimes, I might even need to repeat the renal function in a week, after the patient has been on the NSAID, to make sure there has not been an adverse effect on the kidneys. Also, I may need to closely follow the renal function, if I am upwardly adjusting the dose of the NSAID. There are some patients, where I will not use an NSAID on the basis of their baseline renal function. Conversely, I may need to discontinue an NSAID on the basis of declining renal function.

It is important not to jump the gun when making a decision to discontinue a medication on the basis of an abnormal blood test. If I see a patient is doing well on an NSAID and on a routine surveillance blood screening (to evaluate if the NSAID or other medications on board are adversely affecting any internal organs), I see a new abnormal finding such as decrease renal function, new anemia, or elevation of liver function, the first thing I will do is repeat that blood test. Sometimes blood test results may come back from the lab showing abnormal values and, quite simply put, it may just be a lab error. The last thing I want to do is to disturb the apple cart, but I will, if necessary. It usually takes time to get the patient where I want them to be with regard to adjusting their medications and stabilizing their condition. If they are not having any complaints and their physical exam is stable, I will hold off a day to repeat the test before I make any rash decisions. Conversely, if a patient presents to the office and, on historical and clinical basis I think a medication is causing a problem, I will immediately discontinue the medication, and if appropriate, send the patient to the lab for the necessary blood work.

Aside from potential adverse effects of NSAIDs on the gastrointestinal system and kidneys, this class of medication can also irritate and cause damage to the liver. Consider the liver to essentially be the detoxifying organ of the body. All medications that are absorbed from the gastrointestinal system will circulate through the liver, where most of them will be further broken down into less complex substances. These end products are then delivered through the bile ducts to the intestines for final delivery to the porcelain throne. As you can see, this is not the best medical terminology, but I think you understand the course of directional flow.

NSAIDs, as well as, many other medications, can irritate the liver and cause inflammation of this organ. When the liver enzymes become elevated due to a medication or toxic chemical reaction, such as, by alcohol in large amounts, this is referred to as a "chemical hepatitis." Hepatitis simply means inflammation of the liver. This may, or may not, be a symptomatic process; symptoms can include nausea, vomiting, abdominal pain, fever, anorexia (poor appetite) and in severe cases, jaundice, where the skin and the whites of the eyes turn yellow. Of course, hepatitis also can be caused from various viruses such as hepatitis A, B, C and other viruses. If a patient is on an anti-inflammatory and elevations of the liver enzymes are identified, a careful evaluation needs to be performed to determine the etiology of the liver enzyme(s) elevation. Just because a patient is taking an NSAID and develops elevated liver function tests, one cannot just assume it is because of the NSAID, other etiologies need to be considered, and this may lead to ordering additional investigative studies.

NSAIDs may also have an effect on the central nervous system. These medications may cause mental status changes (especially in elderly patients), tinnitus (ringing in the ears), dizziness and headache. Anti-inflammatories may also be associated with rashes, especially when used in association with excessive sun exposure.

Most NSAIDs can have an impact on bleeding time, which can be associated with an increased potential for bleeding (anywhere). These medications can interfere with the platelet's ability to form a clot after a cut which can be associated with minor or significant bleeding. One particular NSAID called Celebrex does not interfere with platelet aggregation (the process of forming a clot), and hence, this medication is not associated with causing an increased bleeding time (the amount of time needed for a clot to form), as opposed to other NSAIDs. All NSAIDs are associated with an increased potential for bleeding. It is because of the anti-platelet effect of NSAIDs that surgeons insist that patients, who are taking any of these medications, discontinue them 7-10 days before surgery, to minimize the potential for excess bleeding, either during or after a surgical procedure.

Patients who are on blood thinners need to avoid NSAIDs. Celebrex is safe from an increased "bleeding time" potential for the patient on a blood thinner, but even blood thinners have their associated increased risk of causing bleeding. If a patient has a history of a bleeding gastric ulcer and is on the blood thinner Coumadin (warfarin), NSAIDs should not be used. Celebrex could be used in this situation, although many doctors may still not even consider Celebrex as an option in a patient on a blood thinner. Keep in mind, although Celebrex does not affect bleeding time (does not affect platelet aggregation), it still can be associated with similar side effects that are associated with other NSAIDs.

NSAIDs can also be associated with strokes and heart attacks. Patients with a history of heart disease, that take NSAIDs, are at a 13 fold increased risk for developing congestive heart failure, a condition in which the heart is not pumping blood adequately. As a result the lungs can begin to fill with fluid and the lower extremities can retain large amounts of fluid which is called edema. In this situation the patient is usually experiencing fatigue, shortness of breath and possibly chest discomfort.

NSAIDs can also be associated with increased blood pressure. Elevated blood pressure and edema will usually resolve when the NSAID is discontinued. Sometimes to address the edema, it may be necessary to use a diuretic for a short period of time to get rid of the excess fluid. One needs to be careful to discontinue the diuretic once the excess fluid has resolved, since continued use of the diuretic after the NSAID has been withdrawn may cause the opposite effect, dehydration.

As you can see, there are a lot of issues which need to be considered when a decision is made (or not made) to prescribe an NSAID. It is important for the healthcare provider to take a good history from the patient so sound decision making can be accomplished when prescribing an NSAID (or for that matter any medication). I might be very cautious about prescribing an NSAID, to a patient, who is either referred to me or comes on their own depending on the past history, other concomitant medical problems and other medications the patient is taking. If I have a major concern about kidney or liver function, I might even delay initiation of medication therapy for a day or two until I am able to send the patient to the lab to see what their baseline blood work looks like. Once I have that information, I can initiate treatment over the phone. Some patients are not very good historians and can make things more complicated. In that situation, I need to get as much information, as I can, from other doctor records. If not available, I will need to start from scratch. Sometimes in these situations, and I say this with the utmost of respect, it is like practicing veterinary medicine!

Not only is it important for the patient to take medications as prescribed, but also it is very important for the patient to keep their follow-up appointments with their doctor. This is usually not a problem in the early patient-doctor relationship, especially when an accurate diagnosis is in the process of being established and medications are being initiated. Let us fast forward the scenario to where the fibromyalgia or chronic painful condition is under good control and the patient is on a stable medication regimen. In this specific situation, the doctor may want to see the patient at certain set intervals, just to see how the patient is doing clinically, monitor blood work and to refill prescriptions. Patients, who are on chronic opioid medications (narcotics), will need to be seen more frequently than non-opioid patients because of narcotic prescribing guidelines; I will talk more about this later on in the book, when I go over narcotic prescribing.

What the patient needs to understand is the doctor has the responsibility to monitor the patient from many standpoints. The healthcare provider needs to know how the patient is doing. They need to make sure they are not having any problems with the medications being taken. They need to determine whether the medications are still effective at their present doses, if they are still necessary, or whether a dose needs to be adjusted upward or downward. Are there any new problems that may or may not be related to the condition being treated? Are there any side effects from the medications?

It is important to understand the concept: a medication adverse effect can occur at any time during the course of therapy, even years after being on the medication, with no prior adverse effects. Also, I need to know about all the medications being taken, not just the ones which I prescribe. Sometimes, another healthcare provider will put the patient on a medication, without knowing, there may be a contraindication, to taking it with one of the medications I am prescribing. For example, I may have the patient taking an NSAID and then another NSAID was prescribed by a different healthcare provider. One should never take two different NSAIDs at the same time, because this will increase the potential for the various side effects that have already been discussed, which can be associated with the use of even just one NSAID by itself. For patients who take NSAIDs and other medications on a regular basis, the blood work needs to be monitored for abnormalities that might not be clinically evident to the patient, such as, blood loss from the gastrointestinal system resulting in anemia, decreasing renal function, or elevation of liver enzymes.

As a general rule, in a patient who has normal renal and liver function and no history of gastrointestinal bleeding, who I am treating with an NSAID on a regular basis, I am monitoring their blood counts (CBC), every six months; just to make sure all of these parameters continue to remain normal. [Note: CBC stands for complete blood count; this tells me about the hemoglobin level, platelet count and a few other parameters; and the CMP which stands for complete metabolic panel which tells me about kidney and liver function, as well as, electrolyte levels.] In an older patient or a patient who has other medical problems, such as, renal insufficiency, I may need to monitor the blood work more frequently. Of course, if a new situation develops, I may need to repeat blood work immediately. My main point is, just because the patient may be feeling good, they need to keep their follow-up appointment; there are a lot of areas that need to be covered, even if you are feeling well.

Let us talk about some of the various NSAIDs. We will first start by looking at NSAIDs that are available over-the-counter; these medications can be purchased at various places by anybody. A prescription is not necessary. It is important to understand, just because a medication can be obtained (legally or illegally) without a prescription; it does not necessarily mean it is safe for the patient. For example, let us say a patient is told by their healthcare provider they will not prescribe to them an NSAID. [Note: There can be various reasons why an NSAID may be contraindicated for a person; kidney, gastrointestinal, and cardiac reasons to name a few.] NSAIDs, such as, Advil and Motrin (ibuprofen) and Aleve (naproxen sodium) are sold over-the-counter at doses lower than required for prescription strength. A person may not know these are NSAIDs or they may think it is okay to use these medications because, if they are sold over-the-counter and a prescription is not necessary, they must be safe for consumption. This is wrong and clearly not true. If you have been advised you are not to take an NSAID, you should not be using over-the-counter NSAIDs, regardless of their strength.

I do have a pet peeve about the promotion of over-the-counter NSAIDs. In my opinion, there are not enough warnings about their potential adverse effects, even at low doses. I personally believe there should be stronger warnings about these readily available medications. Another thing, to consider, about over-the-counter (OTC) medications, is people tend to take more of the medication than what the directions say on the bottle. As already mentioned, a person should never take two different NSAIDs at the same time because this will significantly increase the potential side effects and adverse reactions that can be associated with the use of even one NSAID.

Sometimes, a person may already be taking an NSAID, prescribed by their physician, and they take it upon themselves to buy an OTC NSAID, because they saw a commercial on TV touting that the product is very effective for pain relief. Ironically, I think it is fair to say, as a general rule, an OTC NSAID will certainly not have the potency and hence, the efficacy of a prescription strength NSAID. If a person, who is already taking a prescription strength NSAID, is not getting the kind of relief that should be achieved, then the decision (by the healthcare provider, not the patient) should be to either increase the dose, if there is room to increase the dose, or to switch to another NSAID. In some particular situations, I may start a patient on an NSAID and tell them to increase or double the dose in a week, providing the problem being treated has not improved, and they are not experiencing any side effect from the medication. Remember, do not take it upon yourself to make any medication adjustments on your own without the direction and approval of your healthcare provider.

Once again, I just want to remind the reader this is not a "how-to" book; my examples are for illustration only. The purpose, of this book, is to empower the patient with regard to their medical care. Of course, you are not going to tell the doctor what to do. However, you can become a greater participant in your own care and be able to bring more to the table with regard to the decision making process of your treatment. There is nothing wrong with asking your healthcare provider if you should make a dose adjustment of the medication, after one week, if there has not been any improvement. Perhaps, there will not be any room to increase the dose. Sometimes, when initially prescribing an NSAID, I will have to put a person on the maximal dose, of the NSAID, because of the severity of the inflammatory process, or on the basis of the patient size. Using NSAIDs, as an example in this case, I will need to give a higher dose to the patient who is 250 pounds compared to the patient who is 150 pounds. With some medications the dose will "not" vary according to weight; the same dose may be appropriate for both the 150 pound and 250 pound person.

OTC ibuprofen comes in the strength of a 200 mg tablet or capsule. Any higher strength of ibuprofen will need to be dispensed with a prescription. The OTC Aleve comes in a 220 mg dose tablet and the directions state not more than two tablets a day are to be taken. As a point of information, Aleve (naproxen sodium) comes in the prescription strength of 375 mg and 500 mg tablets, both which are available in a generic form. Under healthcare provider supervision, there are some patients, who take naproxen sodium up to 1500 mg a day in three individual doses (500 mg up to three times a day). As you can see, there is a big difference between the maximum allocations of OTC Aleve (440 mg per day) versus the prescription strength Naprosyn, with a potential maximal dose of 1500 mg per day. Under strict doctor supervision, the maximal dose of prescription ibuprofen can be as high as 3200 mg per day (800 mg four times a day).

Now, I want to talk about prescription NSAIDs. These medications have been around for decades. Most are available in generic forms, such as, ibuprofen and naproxen sodium which, I have already mentioned. Once I have made the decision that an NSAID is appropriate to prescribe to a patient, I like to present the patient with several medication options. Here is how I break down the options. As a general rule, I look to a generic product, which is how the vast majority of NSAIDs are available. Next, I like to present the patient with an option to take a once-a-day product. Keep in mind, there is a difference between an NSAID which is designed to be dosed truly once-a-day versus an NSAID which is designed to be taken two to three times a day. If an NSAID is supposed to be taken two or three times a day, and is only taken once-a-day, it will probably not be effective as an anti-inflammatory or analgesic (pain reliever) because in order for these medications to work, a certain blood level of the medication needs to be achieved.

The reason, some drugs are dosed once-a-day versus several times a day, is based on the "half-life" of the drug. Simply put, the half-life of a medication is the amount of time needed for half of the dose of the drug to be metabolized. The longer the half-life, the longer it takes for half of the drug dose to be metabolized. If a drug is designed to have a long half-life, it will need to be dosed less frequently. Hence, the once-a-day NSAIDs will have longer half-lives than NSAIDs that have to be taken two to three times a day.

One of the oldest once-a-day NSAIDs is called Feldene (piroxicam). This medication comes in two doses, 10 mg and 20 mg capsules. For most NSAIDs, as a general rule, it takes about five days to achieve the maximal blood level to work as an anti-inflammatory and a few hours to a few days to work as an analgesic (pain reliever). This is why, when you take an NSAID for a swollen painful joint, it will feel better before the swelling fully resolves. If after two weeks, the NSAID has not been effective, I will then consider changing the NSAID. [Note: This decision will depend on the specific condition which is being treated, and also depends upon other medications being taken, as well as, several other factors.]

Another once-a-day NSAID which became generic a few years ago is Mobic (meloxicam). This medication is available in tablet form, 7.5 mg and 15 mg tablets. [Note: The cost of this medication will be the same whether it is prescribed as a 7.5 mg tablet or 15 mg tablet, if purchased using a prescription drug plan.] For my patients that are taking the 7.5 mg tablet, I will ask them if they want me to write for the 15 mg tablet, and they can cut it in half, this way a one month supply will last them two months. If a person does not have insurance and has to pay full tilt at the pharmacy, the 15 mg tablet will cost more but less than two 7.5 mg tablets. If your dose is 7.5 mg a day, then a month of 15 mg tablets (take half a tablet per day) will cost less than two months of 7.5 mg tablets. One word of caution; doing this maneuver will be up to the healthcare provider; it does not hurt to ask. Also, if the desired dose is 7.5 mg and you ask the healthcare provider to write you for the 15 mg tablet make sure that the prescription is not written as 15 mg one half tablet a day, otherwise the pharmacy may give you only 15 tablets since, if the prescription is written that way, 15 tablets at one half tablet a day will only last 30 days.

Another once-a-day NSAID which is available in generic form is Voltaren XR (diclofenac). The non-extended release form of this medication needs to be prescribed in a two to three times a day regimen. The dose for Voltaren XR (the extended release medication) is 100 mg once a day.

Now, we are still keeping with the concept of once-a-day dosing NSAIDs. This next NSAID is called Relafen (nabumetone). This medication is known as a "pro-drug." This has to do with the mechanism by which this medication becomes an active drug. Unlike other NSAIDs, this medication is not active as an NSAID until after it is absorbed and passes through the liver. It is in the liver where this drug is metabolized into its active form. At least in theory, this medication should have less potential to irritate the stomach because it is not an active anti-inflammatory when it "initially" comes into contact with the stomach. Technically, the active form of this medication can come into contact with the surface of the stomach by a process known as "enterohepatic recirculation," which means, after the medication is activated by the liver, it is then secreted into the bile, which is then delivered to the intestines. Once in the intestines, the active medication can move upwards in the gastrointestinal tract to the stomach where it could irritate the lining of the stomach (the gastric mucosa). This medication comes in tablet form and is available in two doses, 500 mg tablets and 750 mg tablets. The maximal daily dose of this medication can go as high as 2000 mg for certain individuals. Although this medication is designed to be a once-a-day medication, the dose can be split, if for example, the medication is working well, but causes some gastrointestinal upset. It is best to take all NSAIDs with some food to help avoid gastrointestinal irritation. This should not be a problem since most people have a harder time refraining from food than taking it, present company included!

The last once-a-day NSAID, I want to discuss, is Celebrex (celocoxeb), noting at this time, there is no generic for this medication. In all likelihood, this medication may be available in generic form in

May of 2014. Celebrex can also be dosed up to twice a day. Celebrex is different from all of the other NSAIDs. As already mentioned, it does not increase bleeding time, which means this medication does not interfere with the process of blood clotting (the time which is necessary for a cut to stop bleeding). I have many patients who are on blood thinners who also take Celebrex; this is safe from the standpoint that Celebrex in and of itself does not increase bleeding time. Keep in mind, there is an increased risk of bleeding in patients on blood thinners. Concomitant use of blood thinners and Celebrex does not "additionally" increase the bleeding time than already is increased with just the blood thinner alone. [Note: All NSAIDs, including Celebrex, can be associated with strokes, heart attacks and a number of other potential side and adverse effects that have already been mentioned.]

Certainly, a patient taking Celebrex also is not immune from developing a gastrointestinal bleed. Many people, who develop gastrointestinal bleeding, are not on NSAIDs or blood thinners. If you have ever seen a late night commercial on TV for Celebrex; it runs about two minutes long. It goes on to explain some of the potential major side effects and adverse reactions that could potentially occur. It is a wonder that anyone would want to take it after hearing about these potential problems. Keep in mind, everything they say regarding adverse reactions can be applied to all NSAIDs. All NSAIDs can be associated with serious problems. All medications have potential side effects. If you were to read the medication profile on Tylenol (acetaminophen) you would never want to take it, too!

NSAIDs which are dosed more than once-a-day are all available in generic form. One important fact to remember is just because a medication is in generic form it is not necessarily inexpensive. With regard to generic NSAIDs, they all do "not" cost the same. If a person has a drug coverage plan from their insurance company, they are well aware of the concept of "tiered" coverage. The tiers may go from 1st (generic), which will be the lowest co-pay. Each insurance plan will have different co-pays for each tier depending upon the plan's coverage benefit, which has been pre-determined by the employer and that particular health plan. The tiers may go from 1st level all the way up to 4th tier. Some medications may not even be available for any type of coverage from the insurance plan, and the patient will be obligated to pay for the entire cost of the medication. In some circumstances, it may be necessary for the doctor to fill out special paperwork so the patient will be allowed to receive that specific medication. In this case, the medication has to be pre-authorized by the insurance company. [Note: If the medication is approved, the patient will still have to pay a co-pay, usually the highest tier co-pay.]

There are plenty of available generic NSAIDs on the market. The vast majority have been around for a long period of time. Already, I have mentioned ibuprofen and naproxen sodium. Others include Trilisate (choline magnesium trisalicylate) and Salsalate (disalcid), both available in 500 mg and 750 mg tablets and usually prescribed on a twice-a-day basis. When I was back in training these two medications were considered the NSAIDs to use when one wanted to prescribe an NSAID which would least likely irritate the gastrointestinal (GI) tract. Another NSAID, which in the past, was felt to be less irritating to the GI tract is Dolobid (diflusinal). This medication comes in a 500 mg tablet and the usual dosing ranges from 500 mg, two to three times a day.

Other commonly prescribed NSAIDs: include Clinoril (sulindac), available in 150 mg and 200 mg tablets usually dosed twice-a-day; Meclomen (meclofenamate) comes in 100 mg tablets and the dosing varies from two to three times a day; Ansaid (flurbiprofen) comes as a 100 mg tablet and the dose can vary from two to three times a day. Voltaren (diclofenac) comes in 50 mg and 75 mg tablets. Already, I have mentioned the availability of Voltaren XR, a 100 mg extended release once-a-day tablet, which is available as a generic product. Usually, Voltaren is prescribed two to three times a day, with a maximum dose of 75 mg three times a day (with food). As a general rule, all NSAIDs should be taken with food to help safeguard the lining of the stomach. Please remember once again, the information, I am giving the reader, is not instructions. Any medication, which is described and discussed in this book, should not be taken without a prescription and specific instructions from their healthcare provider.

Another NSAID that has been around for decades and deserves honorable mention is Indocin (indomethacin). This is a medication that comes in 25 mg and 50 mg tablets. The dose can be prescribed up to three times a day. Special caution should, in my opinion, be taken when prescribing this medication, especially in the older population. This medication can be quite irritating to the digestive tract. Also, this NSAID readily crosses the blood-brain barrier and is more likely to be associated with mental status changes in the elderly. Indomethacin is a classic favorite for doctors to prescribe for patients having an acute gout attack, but other NSAIDs can certainly be used to effectively treat this condition.

Another interesting NSAID that is available (which incidentally has been on the market for over two decades) is a medication called Arthrotec (diclofenac/misoprostol). This is a combination of an NSAID (Voltaren/diclofenac) and a stomach protector (Cytotec/misoprostol). Think of this medication as peanut butter and jelly in one jar. I just went to my refrigerator and took a spoonful of peanut better to eat, I could not help myself! I did however, limit myself to one spoonful! The intended design of this medication is to have an NSAID which is also attached to a separate medication which is used to act as a stomach protector. The misoprostol causes the mucus secreting cells of the stomach to produce more mucus, which in turn gives greater protection to the lining of the stomach from the potentially irritating effect of the NSAID component of the medication (diclofenac). Ironically, it is the misoprostol component of the medication, which often causes GI upset to the point the medication, needs to be discontinued; I personally can attest to this. When this medication first came out, many years ago, we did not have the various types of stomach protectors which we have on the market today, and it was quite an innovative product when it was first introduced. I am not knocking the product as I still have many patients that continue to successfully use this medication.

There is another combination NSAID/stomach protector medication which is called Vimovo. This has been on the market for several years. Vimovo is composed of the NSAID Naprosyn/naproxen sodium and the gastric acid blocker Nexium/esomeprazole.

Certainly, there are several other NSAIDs available on the market. I do think the NSAIDs I have already described are a good representation of what is available and are probably one of the NSAIDs that your healthcare provider is likely to prescribe to you, if an NSAID is needed for either a short or long period of time.

Just remember, there are certain principles which need to be considered when prescribing NSAIDs, either for short-term or long-term use. Healthcare providers may not always have the time to discuss every specific detail or caveat which relates to each medication in the context of each individual patient. Hopefully, the information, in this chapter, will better inform the patient about the specific medications which have been discussed. Remember, it is not my purpose to educate the reader to the extent they go to battle with the healthcare provider. I am trying to empower the reader, so the relationship between the healthcare provider and the patient becomes more of a partnership with a common goal: the patient's healthcare needs. I want to empower the patient so the maximum benefit can be achieved within the allocated period of time the healthcare provider has available for any given visit; whether it is an initial consultation, routine follow-up, or emergency appointment.

SECTION FIVE

Serotonin Specific Reuptake Inhibitors (SSRIs) And Norepinephrine Specific Reuptake Inhibitors (NSRIs)

I now want to talk about a class of medication which, in my experience, has been pivotal with regard to managing fibromyalgia, as well as, a host of other chronic painful conditions, regardless of the etiology of pain; whether its origin is either from degenerative, inflammatory, or neuropathic processes. These medications fall under the class of antidepressants. I have been prescribing them to my patients, with chronic pain for years; they can be very effective in pain management; they also happen to work well for what they were originally designed: the management of depression.

I do not believe a person can be suffering from chronic pain and not experience some degree of depression. I never have seen a person with chronic pain, who initially walks into my office, who is a happy person. It does not mean I will not get them to a happy place. The fact of the matter is, part of the differential diagnosis of fibromyalgia and chronic pain (without any apparent cause, such as, an injury), will include depression. Depressed people hurt. Depression exacerbates pain. Depression can heighten the symptoms of fibromyalgia, and likewise, the pain of fibromyalgia can exacerbate depression. At the end of the day, the patient with either or both depression and fibromyalgia is not a happy camper. The problem, that eventually develops, usually long before they have arrived at my office, is these people are on a vicious merry-go-round, and they need to step off of the ride.

Many patients have a hang-up with the concept of even being depressed. There is a significant amount of patient denial when it comes to the perceived stigma of the diagnosis of depression. Millions of people in the USA and millions of others throughout the world have depression.

I have already discussed antidepressants, which fall under the class of tricyclic antidepressant; amitriptyline, nortriptyline, desipramine and doxepin to name a few. This next class of antidepressant, which I want to showcase, is known as Serotonin Specific Reuptake Inhibitors (SSRIs). The basic mechanism, by which this class of medication acts on the central nervous system, is by increasing the level of serotonin. This hormone has several functions. With regard to chronic pain conditions, the simple concept to remember is the higher the level of serotonin, the less sensitive a person will be to the perception of pain. There may be several working components to the true reason for the effectiveness of these medications in the management of chronic pain; certainly one may be the fact that these medications are antidepressants.

The first SSRI to hit the market in the United States, in 1987, was Prozac (fluoxetine). Although this medication has the FDA indication for the treatment of depression, I have been prescribing this medication to my fibromyalgia and chronic pain patients for many years. This medication can be quite effective for the management of various chronic painful conditions. Usually, this medication is well tolerated. Of course, when you pick up the prescription from the pharmacy, there will be a handout sheet telling you all the "potential" side effects of this medication. I can tell you right now, as with all the other medication handouts, which come along with any filled prescriptions, if you read it, you will not want to take the medication. I really try to discourage patients from reading the medication handouts. Sometimes, patients seem to develop some of the symptoms they read about, probably because they are so concerned about not developing them! Also, just because they are taking a new medication, a new symptom may not necessarily be related to the new medication.

As a general rule, this class of medication will "not" be the first (primary) medication I begin with, in the treatment of fibromyalgia or other chronic painful conditions. I do, however, use SSRIs as part of the medication regimen, when treating chronic pain of any etiology; my philosophy is "pain is pain," regardless of the etiology. It is the etiology of the pain, which may lead me to prescribe one or several drugs over another, but the fundamental concept is: pain needs to be alleviated. Also, experience has taught me, pain can be controlled to "acceptable" levels; the healthcare provider just has to know which medication(s) to use, and more importantly, not be afraid to prescribe what is necessary, and in the appropriate doses to alleviate the pain.

Another issue, there are really no instruction manuals on how to treat chronic pain. Even the management of acute pain is not very well done in general. If you think about it, how can you expect good management of chronic pain when acute pain is often controlled poorly? When I was in medical school, internship, residency and fellowship (1983-1992), I was never given formal training in chronic pain management. Of course, with all fairness to the profession, I did not do formal chronic pain management in my medical training; there are programs in pain management medicine out there. I do not think there is a burning desire for physicians to go into pain management programs; I say this on the basis of the number of physicians (at least in Tucson, Arizona, where I live and have my medical practice) who specialize in pain management. Many rheumatologists make it a point to tell patients up-front, they do not consider themselves to be pain management specialists, and they will not take on narcotic prescribing. Many doctors do not like to take on narcotic prescribing which was started by another physician.

Getting back to SSRIs, I have already mentioned Prozac. If for example, I have a patient with fibromyalgia and their main presenting features are a poor sleep process and widespread pain; I might want first to start that person on 10 mg of Ambien (zolpidem) at bedtime. I will be seeing that patient in two weeks for a follow-up appointment. Keep in mind, I like giving medications a one to two week period of time, to do what they are supposed to do. I will tell you what I would not do. I would not tell the patient to see me in two months for the follow-up appointment. This patient's clinical state, which depends on the response to the medication, will be the same in two weeks as it will be in two months. It will not take two months to get to the desired effect, of the medication (our example here is the patient starting Ambien at 10 mg at bedtime). Two weeks is long enough to know where that patient's response will be to that medication at that dosage. If you find yourself in this situation, where you are prescribed an initial medication, for either fibromyalgia or another chronic painful condition, and are told to come back in 8 weeks, do not bother going back, see someone else. That tells me, and now hopefully you, this healthcare provider does not know how to treat fibromyalgia or chronic pain for that matter.

So, two weeks later, the patient comes back and says they are sleeping better, feels more rested in the morning, but still continues to ache all over, although there has been some improvement overall with the pain; but still experiences pain at an unacceptable level. In this situation, I could consider adding Prozac or one of the other available SSRIs. Remember, Prozac does not have an FDA approved indication, for the treatment of fibromyalgia (this would be another example of the off-labeled use of a medication). As a general rule, you will never run into the problem of needing a medication pre-authorization, from a health plan when filling the prescription of a generic medication when it is being used in an off-labeled fashion. Only the expensive medications are closely monitored by the insurance companies when it comes to off-label prescribing.

When I prescribe Prozac, usually I will start the medication at 20 mg one tablet each morning. The positive effect of this medication, with regard to pain modulation, may take a few weeks. In my experience, when this medication is added to a drug regimen, which already consists of a sleep aid, muscle relaxant and tricyclic antidepressant; the effect of the Prozac may begin within a week, most likely because of the synergistic (additive) effect of the medication combinations. If there has not been any significant response, after two weeks on the 20 mg dose and there have not been any adverse effects with the new medication, I will instruct the patient to increase the dose to 40 mg, to be taken as a single dose in the morning. If there is going to be any significant improvement, on the increased dose of Prozac (40 mg each morning), I would expect the response to be within 2 weeks. If there has not been any significant improvement by that time, that is, less generalized pain, another medication adjustment will need to be made. One possibility would be to increase the dose of the Prozac to 60 mg each morning. The highest dose of Prozac, I will prescribe, to a patient is 80 mg each day. In this situation, with that high a dose, I may split the dose to 40 mg twice a day. Depending upon the residual symptoms, this will dictate the next appropriate medication adjustment or change. The important thing to remember is, "something" has to be attempted, otherwise the present clinical status is as good as it is going to get!

There are several SSRIs which are available that are generic. To be quite honest with you, and based on years of prescribing these medications to patients, they are a good class of safe medications which, for the most part, can be effective equally with pain management, and with treating depression. Prozac has been around the longest and has had the most negative media hype in the past. Several years ago Prozac, which is representative of the SSRI class in general, received a lot of negative publicity. There were reports of increased incidences of suicides in patients, who were taking this medication; this created a new controversy for patients and the medical community. Many physicians have argued, perhaps, it was not specifically the Prozac which was causing the increased suicide attempts, but perhaps because the patient was actually improving by feeling better and having the capacity to take greater initiative; it was this increased capacity which facilitated the process of committing suicide. Simply put, these depressed patients may have lacked the initiative and energy to carry out the act of suicide, but after they were on the Prozac, this medication empowered them to do what they initially were set on doing (suicide).

Unfortunately, depressed people do attempt suicide and some are actually successful. This, of course, is one "theory." Like all medications, one has to weigh the benefits and "potential" risks of taking it. With regard to Prozac, one can certainly argue the case this medication has been helpful for millions of people, who have benefited, throughout the world. All SSRIs have warnings in the package insert about the increased potential for suicidal thoughts and actions, this is nothing new. It should be common practice for healthcare providers to enquire about suicidal thoughts in their depressed patients. Most patients, who have suicidal ideation (thoughts), will not bring it to the physician's attention, but will usually; engage in the conversation, if the question is asked. Of course, this is a sensitive issue and the healthcare provider has to be tactful and sensitive when engaging in this nature of discussion.

While on the topic of suicide, I have had many patients throughout the years who have confided in me, they would have killed themselves had I not been controlling their pain. Chronic pain is not a condition to take lightly. It is very difficult to exist from day to day in a chronic state of pain. I am sure many of my readers can relate to this. I consider chronic, poorly controlled pain a priority to address, this is why I am diligent and aggressive with pain management; relief of pain has not been achieved by the time patients initially see me, and I want to move forward quickly with appropriate and effective management. There is no reason for the suffering to continue. There are enough (generic, low cost) medications on the market to address just about every non-surgical pain out there.

Pain is pain and the perception of a person's pain is relative. When a person comes to my office, for an initial visit, and tells me their pain level is 9 out of 10 (10 being the worst), and by the next visit (usually in 2 weeks), after beginning a new or expanded medication regimen, they tell me their pain is now 6 out of 10; this is real progress. Going from a pain of 9 to 6 is a big improvement; they will even tell you this is progress. This has been a relative and significant improvement on many levels, aside from the actual pain scale. Aside from the improvement with pain, there is a sense of progress which the patient is beginning to see. Many of my patients have been on a long and lonely journey with their pain. Some have been this way for years; having gone to many physicians; having even seen other rheumatologists; and have been to pain clinics in the past, without achieving success with pain management. Even members of my own specialty (other rheumatologists) have varying opinions and perhaps biases when treating chronic pain.

Personalities between the patient and physician are a very important component when treating patients with chronic pain. When a patient finally gets to a doctor, who understands their problem, embraces them as a patient, and then actually makes progress for them after the first visit, there is a new sense of hope which is also a very important process for the patient to experience. This is real progress.

Of course, there has to be mutual patient and physician expectations. I always tell my patients, I am willing to work with them and do my best to help them, but there will not be a cure with one visit. This is going to be a journey which we will take together. Pain is relative; patients know this; and any degree of improvement with pain is always welcomed and creates a sign of encouragement.

Another SSRI is Paxil (paroxetine). This medication comes in 10 mg and 20 mg tablets. I will often initially prescribe this medication at a dose of 10 mg in the morning. The dose can be incrementally increased by 10 mg each week. The maximum dose I prescribe will be 40 mg. There is one point I want to make, sometimes I have observed that psychiatrists may prescribe certain antidepressants at a higher dose than is indicated in the PDR (Physician's Desk Reference). This out-of-the-box prescribing is certainly at the discretion of the psychiatrist. With regard to me, I prescribe many of the antidepressants for fibromyalgia and chronic pain, I am already off-labeling these medications, I will not prescribe any of these medications higher than what the PDR indicates.

Celexa (citalopram) is another SSRI. This medication comes in 20 mg and 40 mg tablets. The starting dose I prescribe is 20 mg. I do have some people taking as much as 60 mg a day of this medication.

Lexapro (escitalopram), which I often refer to as, "the son of Celexa," is available in 5 mg, 10 mg and 20 mg tablets. The 10 mg and 20 mg tablets are scored with a line through the center of the tablet which, when broken in half, will give you two separate halves containing equal amounts of the medication. [Note: If you cut a tablet in half which is not "scored," you will not have equal amounts of the medication within the two halves.] There is also an oral solution (5mg/ml). The starting dose is usually 10 mg with the maximum dose going up to 20 mg each morning. Since the first publication of this book, there is now a generic form of Lexapro on the market.

Another SSRI, which has been on the market for years, is Zoloft (sertraline). This medication is available in 25 mg, 50 mg and 100 mg tablets. The starting dose is usually 25 mg to 50 mg each morning. I have some patients taking up to 200 mg per day of this medication.

I do want to mention one thing at this time (a general statement), about medications that have generics on the market. This is an important concept to understand. A medication may be generic, but certain "doses" of the medication may not be available as a generic. Keep this in mind, if you are prescribed a generic medication and when you get it filled you get sticker shock. This does not happen often, but it does occur. One example, of this phenomenon, is the medication temazepam (Restoril), which I have already mentioned. This medication comes in 7.5 mg, 15 mg and 30 mg capsules. The 7.5 mg capsule does not come in generic form, this will not be inexpensive. Since this is a capsule, it cannot be broken; you just cannot take a half of a 15 mg capsule. Just be aware of this concept.

As a general rule, in my practice, by the time I start prescribing one or two antidepressants (different classes of antidepressants), for my patients, they are usually on several different medications, I am already prescribing for their chronic pain and/or fibromyalgia. I have to use great caution when adding new medications to an already complex medication regimen. Remember, many of these patients have other medical conditions, which are being addressed by other healthcare providers, and they may already be taking several other medications for those conditions. I have some patients, who may be taking in total 15-20 different prescribed medications from their various healthcare providers; even more when you take into account supplemental OTC vitamins, minerals and other products which can be purchased at the drug store without a prescription. I really do not know how these people keep all their medications straight, even with generics on board; all of these co-pays can really add up! Many of my patients tell me they pay as much as $500 a month, just in medication co-pays! This is quite a burden for just about anyone, especially if they are on a fixed income.

The SSRIs which I already have discussed do their thing by one mechanism, increasing the circulating levels of serotonin by blocking the reuptake of serotonin in the brain. It makes sense that by blocking the reuptake of serotonin the level of circulating serotonin increases. Now, as we already know, the SSRIs work differently than other antidepressants, and we also know that for quite some time psychiatrists, pain management specialists and rheumatologists (some rheumatologists do not consider themselves pain specialists and will not treat these patients) have prescribed combination antidepressants to treat depression and chronic pain because each of these medications work on different pathways in the brain. With this in mind, it was only going to be a matter of time until one of the pharmaceutical companies would come up with a medication that would work on two pathways, for example, blocking the reuptake of serotonin and blocking the reuptake of norepinephrine, hence, peanut butter and jelly in the same jar! Now we have several medications available that work in this precise manner. Effexor was the first medication which possessed this "dual modality" mechanism of action (Serotonin Specific Reuptake Inhibitor/Norepinephrine Specific Reuptake Inhibitor, SSRI/NSRI).

Effexor (venlafaxine hydrochloride) is a tablet which comes in several strengths which include 25 mg, 37.5 mg, 50 mg, 75 mg and 100 mg. Also, there is an extended release capsule, which comes in 37.5 mg, 75 mg, and 150 mg doses. The non-extended release Effexor is dosed two to three times a day, with the starting dose usually beginning at 75 mg (in divided doses); the dose can be adjusted to 225 mg per day. Higher doses, of this medication, may be prescribed, usually by a psychiatrist, keeping in mind, in my practice, when I prescribe an SSRI or other antidepressant I am doing it for pain management; I do not prescribe these medications at doses which would be considered outside-of-the-box. The Effexor XR is a once-a-day medication which is taken in the morning, the starting dose is usually 37.5 mg and I have prescribed this medication in doses up to 225 mg per day.

Since the introduction of this dual mechanism other medications of this class have surfaced onto the market. Probably, the most widely known of these dual mechanism antidepressants is Cymbalta (duloxetine). This medication exerts its effect on the central nervous system by blocking the reuptake of serotonin and norepinephrine, two mechanisms of action for the price of one medication, but it is not cheap. There is no generic at this time, but is expected to go generic in 2014. Without medication coverage, this medication will cost too much for the average person. Even with prescription coverage, this will be a high tiered (high cost co-pay), which may still be cost prohibitive to the patient. In some circumstances, a prior authorization may be necessary to obtain this medication for the patient.

It is interesting to note, although there has been a great deal of marketing to the general public and doctor offices about Cymbalta (duloxetine) being approved for the treatment of fibromyalgia, it should be noted this medication has been on the market for several years; its initial FDA indication was for the management of depression. I was off-labeling Cymbalta for years for my fibromyalgia patients and patients with chronic pain. There is a benefit of having a non-generic medication, which does have an FDA indication for the management of fibromyalgia. Sometimes, this high dollar, new medication will be put on the approved insurance plan medication list, but it will be in the most expensive co-pay category. Other times, a prior authorization will be required. In this situation, the insurance company will allow the patient to obtain the medication through the prescription plan providing, it can be documented that a specific protocol was followed. If there are other medications, which are generic and appropriate for the management of the condition, in question, they need to be tried (and failed) first. If the insurance plan does decide to grant a prior authorization, for the new non-generic medication, keep in mind, the patient may have to purchase the medication paying the highest tiered co-pay. Still, it could cost the patient a lot of money. I have seen some insurance companies charge $80 for a high tier co-pay. That is a lot of money to pay a month for just "one" medication!

Cymbalta is available as a capsule in 20 mg, 30 mg and 60 mg doses. I usually start the patient on 30 mg each morning, and usually, I will tell the patient to increase the dose to 60 mg in one week, if tolerated and not improved. If a problem develops, I tell patients to discontinue the medication and notify me without delay. I usually do not prescribe this medication at doses greater than 120 mg each morning, although, I have some patients who are prescribed Cymbalta at higher doses, from their psychiatrists. I think this is a good medication and many of my patients are on this medication as part of their regimen for either fibromyalgia, chronic pain, or both.

Just remember, it is not cheap. For some patients, this may be a therapeutic option which has not been tried. To be quite honest, this is not a medication I would first prescribe, if I have not already used one of the SSRI medications. When effective, patients may derive added pain control while on this medication. Of course, do not forget this medication is an antidepressant and it can be quite effective in treating depression, a component in most patients with fibromyalgia and chronic painful conditions.

There are a few more dual mechanism SSRI/NSRI medications that I would like to mention. They are Savella (milnacipran) and Pristique (desvenlafaxine). Savella, like the others, is an antidepressant which has been around for a long time. What happens is the drug companies are aware that doctors have been prescribing their medications (antidepressants) in an off-labeled fashion for treating fibromyalgia. They then figure out, all they have to do is to design an FDA approved drug study that shows their medication to be safe and effective for the management of fibromyalgia. Keeping in mind, if this is accomplished, the drug will then be given a new FDA approved indication for fibromyalgia; I am simplifying the process! Then the drug companies can target the general public and doctors, and can tout, their drug has been approved, for the treatment of fibromyalgia.

When you think about it, it is a good deal for the pharmaceutical company. They really do know the drug will pass the test in their drug study, because they already know "informally," through conversations with doctors, who have been prescribing their medication off-label, that their drug works. They have plenty of information on how doctors off-label their medication. They already know the drug is safe because people are already taking it for (in this case) depression. The safety studies have already been done for their medication. [Note: However, for the most part, the general public does not know their "new" fibromyalgia drug has already been on the market for years, unless they were already prescribed it, for (in this case) depression. The average person is led to believe this is a brand new product making its debut onto the market. You never see a commercial talking about the "recirculation" of their product!]

I can think of two instances, where a generic medication was recirculated as a brand new product with the associated "non-generic pricing." The first example is Wellbutrin, an antidepressant. It was found that this medication was effective in many patients for the cessation of smoking. I can only assume there must have been observations where people, taking this medication were losing their desire to smoke (obviously a good side effect, except for the tobacco industry). Well, to make a long story short, drug studies were designed to show that Wellbutrin (bupropion hydrochloride) was effective for smoking cessation, and low and behold was the birth (actually rebirth) of Zyban (bupropion hydrochloride). This medication acts on the central nervous system, by weakly blocking the reuptake of norepinephrine, serotonin and dopamine. This is chemically what is happening in the brain when taking this medication; it is, however, unknown how this process exerts its effect on the cessation of smoking, but it is quite effective in many patients, who are eager to quit smoking.

Now, the drug company has the ability (and right) to market this medication to the public and doctors as a new medication with an FDA indication for smoking cessation: this is a true statement. However, this will not be packaged as a generic medication; it will not be cheap. Certainly, patients will pay full tilt for this medication, after all they want to stop smoking for a host of reasons, and if not for anything else, look how much money they will be saving in the long run by quitting smoking. With all fairness to the drug companies, they do spend millions and millions of dollars on the research and development of new products and recirculation of old ones. They are a business, which needs to operate with a positive profit margin. They all have patient assistant programs; doctors are able to treat many of their patients with drug samples furnished from the pharmaceutical companies. People, who work for pharmaceutical companies, are just trying to make a living like everyone else; drug reps all have four year college degrees and often other advanced degrees. I am just stating a fact, about the recirculation of certain medications; it is not my intention to be mean spirited towards the pharmaceutical industry. Remember, it is because of advances, in the pharmaceutical industry we are able to combat many medical illnesses, which allow us to live longer and healthier lives!

The second example of the recirculation of generic medications is our old friend Prozac (fluoxetine). I guess once again, it was observed that women, who were taking this medication and were also experiencing menopausal symptoms, were less symptomatic while taking Prozac. Fast forward to clinical drug studies, which showed indeed, Prozac was beneficial for the management of menopausal symptoms. Of course, Prozac was not going to be reintroduced to the world as "Prozac for menopausal symptoms," certainly; there would not be any money in that. There was also another problem: not many people have warm and fuzzy feelings towards the name "Prozac." Every comedian has told at least one Prozac joke! The average person thinks of Prozac, for depressed people, not to mention having heard something along the way how people commit suicide while taking this medication. Menopausal symptoms can make a woman feel like she is going crazy; but most women do not want to be labeled crazy. Even crazy people do not want to be called crazy! Calling Prozac "Prozac" would have certainly been a problem, even if it did have an FDA approved indication for the management of menopausal symptoms.

Regarding Prozac and the drug company's approach to marketing this medication for menopausal symptoms, the drug company had to come up with a better (less threatening) name for their recirculated product, and they did. I do not know this for a fact, but I "assume" I am probably not far off the mark with my thinking; now I am indemnified (this goes for the Wellbutrin story too). I now introduce to you Sarafem (fluoxetine hydrochloride), Prozac in disguise. Even the name is quite feminine; for heaven's sake half the name is a girl's name (Sara) and fem is short for feminine. Clearly, there was nothing "depressive or crazy" about the naming of this product. Now the PCP or OB/GYN had a medication which was specifically FDA approved for the management of menopausal symptoms, and there was nothing on the surface of this medication that identified it as an antidepressant, "not that there is anything wrong with that,"–TV's Seinfeld episode. I am sure that this must have made office visits with patients with meno-pausal symptoms go much quicker.

Sometimes when off-labeling, a medication (that is, Prozac for menopausal symptoms) there tends to be a lot of salesmanship on the part of the doctor to get the patient to take what they really need. I would never think of off-labeling an antidepressant to a patient with-out reading them the riot act about my intensions for prescribing the antidepressant in an off-labeled fashion. If a patient is prescribed an antidepressant, and they are not aware, they are getting an antidepres-sant to be used in an off-labeled way; the healthcare provider needs to be prepared to get an angry phone call from the patient. Shortly after the prescription leaves the hand of the patient, the pharmacist will be informing the patient their new medication is an antidepres-sant. [Note: It will not be the pharmacist who will be explaining the off-labeled use of the medication to the patient. It is also quite pos-sible, the pharmacist may not be aware of the off-labeled use of the medication.] I have had more than one phone call from a pharmacist, in the past, enquiring about my intended use of a medication I was prescribing, in an off-labeled fashion, mostly because of the confusion which was created by not fully explaining to the patient the off-labeled use of the medication. I have not had these phone conversations in many years because I have learned, what is necessary to explain to the patient, to avoid this type of confusion. The prescribing doctor also has to be careful when giving a prescription, to a patient, which is to be used in an off-labeled manner. The patient may do their own research, before even turning the prescription in, at the pharmacy, and when they see there is no mention of the medication having an indication to treat their condition, the patient may come to the immediate conclu-sion you do not know what you are doing and decide to not come back for a follow-up appointment.

Getting back to the combination SSRI/NSRI medications, Savella and Pristique fall into this class of medication. Savella actually has an FDA indication for the management of fibromyalgia. [Note: Its origi-nal indication was for depression.] This medication comes in doses of 12.5 mg, 25 mg and 50 mg tablets. The starting dose is 12.5 mg (this medication actually comes in a starter pack with 12.5 mg, 25 mg and 50 mg tablets). The maximal dose is 100mg twice a day.

Pristique is another member of the SSRI/NSRI family. At the present time, this is a medication, which is FDA indicated for the management of depression. To prescribe this for the management of fibromyalgia and chronic pain would be to do so in an off-labeled fashion. I do have some patients on this medication, but it is being prescribed by their psychiatrist for depression. I certainly do not know this medication well, but I suspect it may prove helpful in an off-labeled fashion for the management of fibromyalgia and chronic pain. I see no reason why Pristique should not be helpful, in those conditions, since the other medications of the SSRI/NSRI class have already proven themselves (at least to me) to be effective and helpful for these painful conditions. Remember, a doctor can write a script for any of these medications; whether they feel comfortable doing so (when off-labeling) is another story.

In my opinion, through my years of experience, the only way to achieve successful pain management for the fibromyalgia patient is to think and practice in an off-labeled, outside-of-the-box manner. When I see a patient with fibromyalgia, I am not thinking about FDA approved drugs. At this point in time, the only FDA approved drugs, for the treatment of fibromyalgia are Lyrica (I have not gone into detail on this medication, yet), Cymbalta and Savella; this is the chronologic order of the FDA's approval for these medications for the management of fibromyalgia. [Note: All of these drugs have been on the market for many years with FDA indications to treat other conditions.]

Lyrica was the first drug to get FDA approval for the management of fibromyalgia; this indication was granted in 2007. I have been successfully treating fibromyalgia for over 20 years; how did I ever get by without Lyrica, or Cymbalta, or Savella for all of these years? The answer, off-labeling! In my opinion, if there were never any new drugs, which came out on the market for the specific management of fibromyalgia, the world of fibromyalgia would survive and do quite well. There are plenty of available medications for the management of fibromyalgia, most are generic, and you just have to have a doctor who is willing to prescribe them. The problem is most healthcare providers do not know what to do for fibromyalgia. It is hard enough for them to make the diagnosis. Then, on top of all of this, to prescribe a medication in an off-labeled fashion is going to put the average healthcare provider way out of their comfort zone. The patient, as well as, the practitioner become mutually frustrated, unfortunately, the patient continues to be in pain and the healthcare provider moves on to their next patient.

SECTION SIX

Anti-Seizure Medications

This next class of medication is rather interesting, in how it fits into the management of fibromyalgia and chronic pain. I specifically want to talk about four medications in particular. Interestingly enough, they fall into the class of an "anti-seizure" medication. These medications have been extremely helpful, to my patients, with fibromyalgia and chronic pain. You may already be asking the question, how does this work?

Let us discuss the mechanisms by which painful impulses are perceived in the brain. I will keep this very simple. We experience pain because we have a central nervous system which tells us we are in pain. For this to occur, there are complex biochemical reactions which occur in the peripheral and central nervous system. One way of trying to treat pain would be to interrupt this transmission process, which tells the brain we are experiencing pain. Several anti-seizure medications, especially the four, which I am about to review, slow down the transmission to the brain of pain impulses, thereby, treating the chronic pain.

I explain the mechanisms of action of these drugs, to my patients, by stating, these medications act as volume control dials; they have the capacity to turn down the pain "volume." Yes, this is not very scientific, but do you really care? All I can say is, I have been prescribing these medications, to my fibromyalgia and chronic pain patients for years, and they have been quite effective, doing exactly what I tell the patient they will do for them; turning down the "volume" (intensity) of the pain.

The first of these four medications, I will present to you, is a drug called Neurontin (gabapentin). This is a medication which has been around for years. Aside from its value as an FDA approved anti-seizure medication, I have been off-labeling this medication for years to my fibromyalgia and chronic pain patients. This medication is quite helpful for people who suffer from painful neuropathies; diabetic neuropathy is common; as are, neuropathies from many etiologies, such as, certain vitamin deficiencies; chemotherapy, radiation therapy, phantom pains (where a person has had a limb amputated, and they still perceive pain where that limb used to be), and nerve pain due to trauma or from an arthritic process which impinges on nerves.

It should make sense to understand that pain is not necessarily associated with inflammation, so NSAIDs are not always helpful, especially when the pain is neuropathic. Remember, an NSAID may be helpful with a painful non-inflammatory condition by virtue of the fact these medications also function as analgesics (pain relievers). Sometimes, there may certainly be value for the use of an NSAID along with Neurontin for pain management. When one uses more than one medication for the management of any painful condition; there has to be consideration to the etiology of the pain and, at least in theory, the mechanisms and pathways, which need to be blocked to effectively address the pain.

There is usually more than one mechanism involved which mediates the pain process, hence, the rationale for combination drug therapy, for the management of fibromyalgia and other chronic painful conditions. As a general rule, this class of medication is not the first drug I use when building a pain management regimen for my patients. As I have already mentioned, sleep disturbance is a fundamental problem for many of my patients with chronic pain. I like to start things off with a sleep aid. Keep in mind, although I generally do not like to begin with more than one medication, when attempting to build a chronic pain management medication regimen, there will be situations when I will start a patient on more than one medication at a time. It depends on what is going on at the time of the visit. However, it would not be uncommon for me to start off by giving a patient a sleep aid, an NSAID and a muscle relaxant, providing each medication is appropriate in treating the presenting symptoms.

Later on in the book (after I have given the reader a basic foundation regarding my approach to treating fibromyalgia and chronic pain), I present real clinical cases, which I have been successfully managing for years. After I have laid down the groundwork for treating patients, with these conditions, you will be able to follow my rationale for how I make a diagnosis and the approach to medication management for these conditions. I feel quite confident the reader will be able to associate themselves with one or more of my case presentations. This is for the purpose of illustrating to the patient, they are not alone with their specific painful condition, but more importantly, there is effective, inexpensive treatment for the condition for which they have been suffering, oftentimes for many years.

The purpose of this book is to empower the reader, who suffers from fibromyalgia and chronic pain. To give them the ability to better understand their condition; and most importantly, seek out the appropriate healthcare professionals that will afford them the greatest help. My philosophy is; nobody deserves to suffer. People who have chronic pain never asked for it, they all want it to go away. Sadly, chronic pain does not go away by itself; that is why it is called "chronic." However, chronic pain does not mean you have to chronically suffer. The vast majority of my patients, who suffer from chronic pain, are not doing much suffering once I have gotten them on their custom tailored pain regimen.

Getting back to Neurontin, this is a medication I like to prescribe to patients, who ache all over, experience generalized pain and suffer from fatigue. The value of this medication is derived when I add it to the sleep aid. Oftentimes, I am able to correct the sleep disturbance with one of the sleep aids I have previously mentioned, but the patient continues to experience pain. I have had great success with the use of Neurontin in this situation. Remember, I am off-labeling this medication when I prescribe it for the management of fibromyalgia or other painful conditions. I have also found this medication to help with the sleep process either in combination with a sleep aid or by itself. This medication is usually prescribed three times a day, and I specifically tell the patient to take the last dose right before going to bed. Also, I have found this medication to be helpful for many patients, who have nighttime muscle cramps and restless leg syndrome. In these situations, I may prescribe the Neurontin to be taken only at bedtime.

I have mentioned several situations where Neurontin has been helpful to treat conditions in which there is no FDA indication for the use of this medication, for example, fibromyalgia, chronic painful conditions, restless leg syndrome, nocturnal (nighttime) muscle cramps and insomnia. I also have patients, who benefited from Neurontin, who experience chronic headaches. I have found this medication to be key ammunition in the arsenal of drugs which successfully combats fibromyalgia and other chronic painful conditions. It is available in generic form; is tolerated well by most patients; and, has the ability not to interfere with other medications the patient already may be taking for the management of other medical conditions. Neurontin (gabapentin) is available in 100 mg, 300 mg, 600 mg and 800 mg tablets. Some manufacturers make the medication in capsule form. The advantage of the tablet is: it can be broken so incremental dose adjustments can be attained. In an elderly patient or a patient who relates a history of medication sensitivity at low doses, usually, I will start the dosage of Neurontin at 100 mg three times a day (last dose to be taken before bedtime) with instructions to double the dose (two 100 mg tablets three times a day) in one week, if the medication has been tolerated and there has not been any improvement. I then see the patient in two weeks, for a follow-up appointment, and further management will be contingent on the patient's response to the medication.

For other patients, I will start the Neurontin at 300 mg three times a day (last dose to be taken at bedtime) also instructing the patient to double the dose (two 300 mg tablets to be taken three times a day) after one week, if the medication is tolerated and they are not improved. I will be seeing the patient two weeks later for the follow-up appointment and further management will be contingent on how the patient responded to the medication. When a patient comes back after two weeks, and tells me the medication was well tolerated, but they feel no different, I will then increase the dose, usually to 300 mg three times a day to the patient whose dose was up to 200 mg three times a day and 900 mg three times a day to the patient, who was up to 600 mg three times a day. I will not consider this medication to be a failure unless the patient has reached the maximal dose (3600 mg per day), providing there are no side effects, along the way, as the dose of this medication is increased.

Another medication, which falls under the anti-seizure family, which I have found to be quite helpful for my fibromyalgia and chronic pain patients, is Topamax (topiramate). Like Neurontin, this medication does not have an FDA indication for fibromyalgia nor chronic pain, but I have prescribed this medication to numerous patients with these conditions noting, this medication has been quite effective for many of these patients. Also, many of my patients with fibromyalgia suffer from migraines; Topamax can be very helpful in addressing migraines in my patients with fibromyalgia, especially if migraines are a significant symptom they experience. It only has been in the past several years, or so, that Topamax has been available as a generic medication; since this time, I have been prescribing this medication in increasing numbers because it is now very affordable.

Remember, when this medication was not in a generic form, I was not able to get this authorized for my fibromyalgia and chronic pain patients because without an FDA indication, the insurance companies would not approve the use of this medication. Once a medication becomes generic, insurance companies do not know, nor do they care why the patient is using the medication! Topamax is a favorite, for many of my patients, because of one of its most common side effects, weight loss (yes, I said weight loss)! This is in contrast to Neurontin, which has the potential of causing weight gain (not very often). My larger patients love it when Topamax is one of the medications in the offering, when I review the four anti-seizure medications which they could possibly use. I have had patients who, without trying, have lost as much as 50 pounds over 6 months on Topamax.

I understand how difficult it is for people to lose weight, especially if they suffer from chronic pain; it is difficult to even move around the house let alone getting minimal amounts of exercise. Many patients with chronic pain are depressed, one of the only pleasures they have left may be to eat (usually not healthy stuff either). As a result, many of these patients are overweight, Topamax is like a dream drug for some of these patients; it addresses their fibromyalgia and/or chronic pain, "possibly" assists with weight loss, and is generic to boot; the only thing that could make it better would be if it was free and came with a Hot Fudge Sundae!

Because of the potential for significant weight loss, I am very cautious when prescribing this medication to thin people; some of my patients cannot afford to get any thinner. Topamax is available in 25 mg, 50 mg, 100 mg and 200 mg tablets. I usually will start a patient out at 25 mg twice a day with the instruction to increase the dose to 50 mg twice a day in one week, if tolerated and not improved. Their follow-up appointment will be in two weeks, and at that time I will review their progress and determine what the next step will be. Usually, I will adjust the dose upwards to as high as 200 mg twice a day, if needed. It is always going to be a judgment call, on my part, as to how far I will go with a medication for my patients; whether it is labeled or off-labeled prescribing. I always tell the patient, when I am going to prescribe to them a medication, which will be used in an off-labeled fashion. I almost never have a patient object to the off-label prescribing of a medication.

It is all about communication with the patient. My patients are quite happy I am doing "something" for them. I always tell them, if they walk into the office and are experiencing pain on their present medication regimen, no matter how long the visit takes, it will mean nothing unless the patient leaves the office with a medication dose adjustment, a new prescription, or a plan to address the pain using a non-medication modality, such as, physical therapy in the appropriate patient. Do not misunderstand my intentions. I am not out to put the world on medications. I just know how to cut to the chase, and I know what people who wind up at my office really need. By the time they get to me, they have been through the mill with doctors; I tell them the buck stops here!

Similar to Neurontin, Topamax in most circumstances will not be the first drug I pull off the shelf. Topamax, as with Neurontin, is usually my "add to" medication. The patient will most likely be on a sleep aid and possibly an NSAID or even a muscle relaxant before I add one of the anti-seizure medications. Just keep in mind, there is no cookbook on how to manage fibromyalgia or chronic painful conditions; this adds to the complexity of treatment. You need a doctor, who has a lot of experience (trailblazing) with these conditions, to be effectively managed. Unfortunately, there is a "Catch 22" to this whole process. It is like a person graduating from college who applies for a job, but they are told they are not qualified because they do not have practical experience. On the other hand, there may be a person doing a job, who has no opportunity for upwards mobility because they may not have the college degree. The chronic pain specialist has to start somewhere. Nobody wants to be an experiment. All I can say is, I have made that journey from the mailroom to the boardroom; I have always had the best intentions for my patients and today, I owe what I know, to them.

Another anti-seizure medication that I want to mention is the very well-publicized Lyrica (pregabalin). [Note: There is, at this time, no generic available for Lyrica.] Lyrica has the distinguished honor of touting itself as the first FDA approved medication for the management of fibromyalgia. Just remember, this medication was not originally designed to treat fibromyalgia, it was already on the market for several years and got an additional FDA indication, after the drug company Pfizer did a few controlled drug studies using Lyrica for the management of fibromyalgia. Lyrica's first FDA indication was for the management of a specific type of seizure. Interestingly enough, Lyrica has three other FDA approved indications, other than for the treatment of fibromyalgia: certain seizure disorders in adults, diabetic peripheral neuropathy and post herpetic neuropathy (a condition which is associated with pain over the region where a person previously had a viral infection called Varicella Zoster (Shingles).

For years, I was off-labeling the use of Lyrica for my fibromyalgia patients, and patients with various chronic painful conditions. Before the FDA's approval of Lyrica for the management of fibromyalgia, most of my patients, who were taking it, were on samples I was able to give them because the drug company would furnish me with an endless supply. Before Lyrica was approved, by the FDA, for the management of fibromyalgia, most insurance companies would not approve the use of Lyrica for this condition; the patient was out of luck, unless I had a sample to give to them. Now, with Lyrica having the FDA indication for fibromyalgia, it is easier to prescribe this medication for patients. The biggest problem with this medication is, it is expensive, and will be a high tier co-pay for the patient. Some insurance companies will only approve the medication if a few other generic medications have been tried and failed. Funny how you have to have failed a few generic non-FDA approved medications for the treatment of fibromyalgia before they will let you have the FDA approved medication (Lyrica). Certainly, there is no love lost here between the patient and the insurance company.

In my opinion, however, if a doctor thinks Lyrica is going to be the ultimate medication for the management of fibromyalgia, they are not going to get too far with treating this condition by prescribing only Lyrica. Remember, in my opinion, the fundamental problem in patients with fibromyalgia is, they have an abnormal sleep pattern, which sets the stage for all the other features of this condition. This is why the first thing, which has to be done with these patients, as I have mentioned previously, is to address the abnormal sleep pattern; Lyrica does not do this. A patient, who is given Lyrica as their initial treatment may feel a bit better, but they are not going to get too far regarding the abnormal sleep process. This is why many patients, who are only prescribed Lyrica as a single therapy agent do not do well. This becomes quite frustrating for both patient and physician because, when this fails they do not know what to do next. The promoters of Lyrica have created great expectations for this medication in the management of fibromyalgia; for doctors, who only prescribe medications by the book (the PDR – Physician's Desk Reference), soon they will feel lost when Lyrica has failed. Of course, they may now turn to Cymbalta or Savella (antidepressants that were assigned the additional FDA indication for the treatment of fibromyalgia). Keeping in tune with my philosophy of the approach to fibromyalgia, I would not prescribe any of these three medications (Lyrica, Cymbalta, nor Savella) as any "initial" treatment for the management of fibromyalgia.

When Lyrica received its FDA indication for the management of fibromyalgia, I found it rather interesting (and frustrating) because the pharmaceutical company which makes the medication (Pfizer) had a massive "direct to the public" campaign of their "new product" (wink, wink), Lyrica, the first FDA approved medication for the management of fibromyalgia. For the first time on television, this orphan condition of fibromyalgia finally had a home with its very own "new" medication (Lyrica), even though it had been on the market for years for the management of a few other FDA approved conditions, which I have already mentioned.

My biggest concern, with this type of direct-to-patient marketing, was the general public was hearing about this "new" fibromyalgia drug in advance of the prescribing physicians, who did not have a good understanding of how this medication was supposed to be used for the management of fibromyalgia. I had discussions with other doctors who told me, their patients were either calling them or asking them at their office appointments to put them on Lyrica for their fibromyalgia. Considering that a fair number of doctors, do not even believe that the condition exists, you can only imagine the position doctors were in with the direct marketing to the public with this medication. If anything, I think this approach created more confusion about the recognition of fibromyalgia and its treatment. Perhaps, this was well calculated by the drug company, by having patients directly approach the doctor for the specific advertised treatment. However, doctors tend not to prescribe medications they are not used to prescribing; many doctors do not want to be the first to prescribe a new medication.

This created a complex set of circumstances. Patients with fibromyalgia needed treatment. Of course, the pharmaceutical company wanted to promote and sell their product; I still take the stand that doctors (as a general rule) want what is best for their patients; I just think, in this situation, there was a disconnect between the drug company, the doctor and the patient. At this point in time, however, it is a moot point. Enough time has passed, everyone now has heard of fibromyalgia; and doctors are giving greater recognition to this condition, mostly because there are FDA approved medications available for this mysterious and poorly understood, yet very prevalent condition. However, I do think doctors are being misguided on how to treat fibromyalgia. I am not saying the drug companies are conspiring; they are capitalizing just on the fact they have FDA indications for their drugs for the management of fibromyalgia.

The drug reps will attempt to educate the doctors about fibromyalgia in the context of their product. There is nothing wrong with this; I just do not feel these three medications with FDA indication for the management of fibromyalgia (Lyrica, Cymbalta and Savella) are the best choices as "initial" therapy for the management of fibromyalgia. Remember, these medications do not come in generic form and will cost more than a generic product. I do have many patients on each of these medications and, with all honesty; I have had great success with each of them. [Note: As with other medications they certainly do not work in all patients.]

I only can say, in my experience with each of these FDA approved products, I have not had much success when they are used as a single drug therapy for my fibromyalgia patients. Sometimes, I will even have patients taking combinations of Lyrica and Cymbalta, or Lyrica and Savella. I would not combine Cymbalta and Savella because they are both SSRI/NSRI medications (antidepressants). I have found each of these medications to be helpful for chronic pain syndromes of multiple causes. Pain is pain. The brain interprets discomfort. These medications are effective in turning down the volume of pain which is interpreted in the central nervous system. Do not forget, two of these medications have their foundations in the management of depression (Cymbalta and Savella), and they can be very effective antidepressants [Note: Addressing depression may also be an important component in the management of chronic pain.] Certainly, pain can exacerbate depression and vice versa. The majority of my fibromyalgia and chronic pain patients take an antidepressant as a component of their medication regimen.

Lyrica is available as a capsule. It comes in several doses, 25 mg, 50 mg, 75 mg, 100 mg, 150 mg, 225 mg and 300 mg. This medication is dosed two to three times a day. The usual starting dose is 50 mg - 75 mg two to three times a day. Sometimes, even at these low doses, a patient may experience drowsiness and lethargy; when this occurs, I will usually instruct the patient to decrease the dose to one tablet in the morning and stay at that dose for a week before increasing the dose back to the original starting dose. Just keep in mind; sometimes people experience side effects to even entry level doses of medications. If every medication was discontinued each time a minor side effect developed (especially when initially starting a new medication) you would be going through different medications left and right. Most of the time, all that is necessary to do in these situations, is to cut the dose back and give the body about a week to get used to the new medication. I always tell the patient, when I cut the dose down in these situations, they are probably not going to experience a positive clinical response at the lower dose; that should occur after the body "adapts" to the medication and with higher doses.

A medication has to be tolerated before it has the ability to be effective at a therapeutic dose. As with just about every medication, which is used in the management of fibromyalgia and other chronic painful conditions, the effective dose of the medication(s) on board will need to be titrated (adjusted) to achieve the maximal benefit from any specific dose. Lyrica is no different. If you look at the Lyrica drug studies, it was determined that the maximal effective dose for the management of fibromyalgia is 450 mg per day in two to three divided doses. For some conditions, which are FDA approved for the use of Lyrica, the maximal dose of this medication is 600 mg per day. The clinical trials have shown that fibromyalgia patients did not benefit from doses higher than 450 mg per day. Well, in my medical practice, I have many patients who do not respond to 450 mg per day of Lyrica; but do very well on 600 mg per day. In these situations I am "dosage" prescribing "outside-of-the-box." Keep in mind, if you are taking Lyrica, from a prescriber, who, if strictly dosage prescribing by the book (the PDR), you might get short changed if you are taking Lyrica at a dose of 450 mg per day and not achieving a maximal response from the 450 mg per day dose. Remember, the response to a medication is going to be dose dependent. In my book (literally), a patient is not a Lyrica failure unless they have taken the drug at 600 mg per day and they have tolerated the medication without any significant positive response. One of the more common side effects is some patients may tend to gain weight on this medication; the opposite of what one usually sees with Topamax.

One final anti-seizure medication which I have given patients for the management of various types of painful conditions is called Lamictal (lamotrigine). This medication has an FDA indication for the treatment of certain types of seizure disorders and certain patients who have bipolar disorder. Keep in mind, when I prescribe Lamictal, I am doing so in an off-labeled manner. One of the serious potential side effects of this medication is it can be associated with a very severe life threatening skin rash condition. In the management of seizure disorders, the maintenance dose of this medication varies between 200mg - 400mg per day. When initiating this medication, the starting dose should be 25mg and slowly titrated upwards to the desired effective dose by a healthcare provider who is experienced with the use of this medication.

SECTION SEVEN

Stimulants

Switching gears a bit, with regard to medications which are used to treat fibromyalgia, I have found the class of medications known as "stimulants" to be extremely effective in managing the fatigue associated with fibromyalgia and chronic painful conditions. [Note: These will all fall under the category of off-labeling.]

There are several stimulants on the market, some have generic forms. As a general rule, I never use these drugs as initial treatment, unless the patient has fatigue as the only complaint. Fatigue is a key and fundamental problem which many patients experience, with or without fibromyalgia. It is not uncommon for depressed patients to feel fatigued. Obviously, in the depressed patient, the depression has to be addressed. You may have heard of some of these medications, such as, Adderall (dextroamphetamine), a medication which is widely prescribed to the pediatric population for attention deficit and hyper-activity disorders.

The value, of a stimulant, is it helps the patient to be more alert, stay focused, and feel more energized. They are to be taken first thing in the morning, and the dosing should be either a single dose or possibly divided to morning and noontime dosing; every patient will differ on their response to the timing and dosage of stimulants. Remember, the concept is to take the medication in the morning so it promotes energy for the rest of the day. You would not want to take this medication in the evening or at night, unless you are a shift worker and night-time is your daytime. If you take it at night, you will never get to sleep.

When you think about it, one would think there would be a big dilemma with regard to treating a patient, with a stimulant, who already has a sleep disturbance. Would not prescribing a stimulant, to a patient, who already cannot sleep make the sleeping problem worse? You would think the last thing these insomniacs need is a medication designed to wire-up the patient. The fact of the matter is, in the right setting, a stimulant is a perfect and appropriate medication to give to some patients, who experience severe fatigue. There are several concepts to bear in mind, when looking at the rationale behind giving a patient a stimulant. First, when a patient wakes up in the morning and is totally exhausted, this is a big problem. When we wake up we are supposed to be rested so we can set out on our mission of the day, whatever that may be. Waking up tired is not a good start; things are only going to get worse as the day progresses.

Second, I want to focus on the example of a patient, who has fibromyalgia, not sleep apnea, a common cause of chronic fatigue, and whose sleep process and pain issues have been managed with a few medications. We have taken the journey to the point where all that is really prevalent is the patient's chronic fatigue. Remember, if the patient can sleep well; feel rested in the morning; especially with appropriate medication management; but still experience debilitating fatigue, that is where the role of the stimulant comes into play. Some patients will describe fatigue, which is present as soon as they wake up. Others will say they do okay for a few hours in the morning, but then the fatigue sets in, and they are done for the day by noon. Everyone is different, but there are common threads to the fatigue process, and the concept of treating these patients will be the same, a stimulant is needed.

I have one quick statement on the topic of stimulants. This is a class of drugs, which many healthcare providers will not feel comfortable prescribing. I know of many, who have never prescribed any of them to their patients. I have already discussed the process of writing medications for the management of fibromyalgia and chronic painful conditions in an off-labeled manner. Many healthcare providers, however, do not feel comfortable treating a condition, with a medication which does not have an FDA indication. Between the off-label prescribing of medications; writing for stimulants which are not FDA approved for chronic fatigue; and the use of another class of medications, which I have not reviewed yet (narcotics); you can see why it is difficult for patients with fibromyalgia and chronic painful conditions to get appropriate management. For a doctor who thinks and prescribes outside-of-the-box, it will have taken a long time (years) for the practitioner to be proficient and savvy with treating these conditions.

One of the stimulants on the market for many years is Adderall, an amphetamine. As already stated, this is a medication, which is widely used in the pediatric population for the treatment of ADD/ADHD (Attention Deficit Disorder/Attention Deficit Hyperactivity Disorder). This is a medication, which I often prescribe, to patients, who experience chronic fatigue and excessive daytime drowsiness. This is a generic medication, which comes in various doses. I will prescribe this medication as a once-a-day drug to be taken after getting up in the morning. I will usually start the patient on a 10 mg tablet and will see the patient in two weeks for a follow-up appointment. The patient's response will determine additional dose adjustments at subsequent office appointments. There are a few precautions, which I will discuss with the patient at the time of prescribing this medication. These medications, for the most part, are well tolerated by patients. Sometimes they can be associated with an accelerated heart rate and agitation. There are a host of other potential side effects, but the bottom line is, it is unusual for me to have to discontinue stimulants because of a side effect, in patients, I treat with chronic fatigue issues.

Stimulants are controlled substances. What this means to the patient is, when you are prescribed one of these medications, a new prescription will be required to present to the pharmacist each time the medication needs to be refilled. The doctor is not able to write for refills on that specific script. This means the doctor will have to write separate scripts, if he or she wants you to have refills of the medication. In this situation, if multiple prescriptions of the same controlled substance are given to the patient, at one office visit, for patients, who are on chronic and stable medication regimens, each prescription must have on it the date that it was written, and the date that it is able to be refilled. [The ability of the physician to write prescriptions in this manner may vary from state to state.] This is an indication to the pharmacist that the prescription is not to be filled before a certain time period. [Note: Typically, one month after the prior same medication prescription was written.] This is to ensure patient compliance with filling a controlled substance prescription. If multiple prescriptions were written, for the same patient, with the same date on each prescription without additional filling instructions, on the prescription, for the pharmacist, a patient could conceivably take each prescription to separate pharmacies on the same day and then have multiple prescriptions filled. The doctor has to safeguard the patient (and themselves) from getting into trouble. This is a common practice I employ when writing scripts (prescriptions) for controlled and sometimes non-controlled, substances.

As a general rule, whenever I prescribe a new controlled substance, I will only write one script for that medication (initially); for many reasons. It would not be appropriate for me to give more than one script for a new controlled medication. Why would I do that, when there is the potential this medication may not be tolerated and would need to be changed? As a prescriber of a controlled substance, I have to be concerned about the final destination of that medication and any scripts I write. If I gave a person two new scripts (sequential scripts of the same medication) and two days later, I get a phone call telling me, they had a side effect from that medication; there is an expectation I will be giving them a new script for another medication. In all likelihood, the patient will need another controlled substance to replace the medication they are not tolerating. At this point in time, not only do they have almost a full month of the new controlled medication (and an extra prescription), but I now have to prescribe a new medication. From my end of things, this could give a pharmacist the impression I am indiscriminately prescribing controlled substances. This could potentially result in a complaint to the DEA (Drug Enforcement Agency) and I could be at risk of losing my license to prescribe narcotic medications; this would certainly be the end of my medical career! Also, this could potentially involve (in my state) the Arizona Board of Medical Examiners, resulting in a host of problems which could vary from a slap on the wrist, to loss of my medical license; the latter would be a career ender.

It is somewhat of a touchy situation when I prescribe controlled substances for patients. I need to be convinced (in my mind) a controlled substance is appropriate for that patient. I always want to see that patient in two weeks to see how they have responded to the medication. I may need to increase the dose at the next visit or possibly change to a new medication, if it has not been tolerated. It will be a judgment call on my part, when I feel comfortable giving multiple (same medication) sequential controlled substance prescriptions to a patient. My rule is I will give 2 to 3 consecutive scripts, for a controlled substance, once I have the problem at hand controlled on a specific medication at a specific dose, and this could involve multiple different medications. These are usually my chronic pain patients, who I have been treating for a long time, and mutual trust has developed between the patient and me. I trust the patient to take their medication as pre-scribed and on schedule; and the patient trusts me, knowing I will give them what is needed to effectively manage their painful condition.

An interesting phenomenon, I have observed throughout the years, is when a patient comes to see me and tells me their doctor decided they no longer need pain medications; and they are no longer going to prescribe them to that patient anymore. The first thing I now have to do, is to determine if the patient is drug seeking, or is it appro-priate for continued use of the controlled substance; perhaps needing even higher doses or expansion of controlled medication therapy. The bottom line is the vast majority of patients with chronic pain need to be on a medication regimen; the pain is not going to go away on its own. It is not called chronic pain for nothing. When a patient comes to me and tells me they have been suffering from chronic pain for several years, in spite of being on a chronic pain regimen, my approach has to be to "change something," what is on board is certainly not working and something new has to be done. Sometimes, the "something new" involves only increasing the dose of one or more medications already on board; sometimes I have to make major (yet incremental) changes in the medication regimen. I will talk more about this approach, when I review (later in the book) the various narcotics I prescribe for certain patients, who suffer from chronic pain.

Getting back to the class of stimulants, another medication, which I like to prescribe, is Metadate CD (methylphenidate hydrochloride). As with Adderall, this medication is taken as a single dose in the morn-ing. The initial starting dose is 10 mg; I have some patients who take single daily doses as high as 60 mg each morning.

Provigil (modafinil) is another medication which is a stimulant. This medication became generic in 2012. The starting dose is between 100 - 200 mg each morning. The maximal dose is 400 mg each morning.

Another stimulant, which is on the market, one of the newer ones with no generic form, is a medication called Nuvigil (armodafinil), similar to Provigil (modafinil). To be quite honest with you, I have never prescribed Nuvigil to any of my patients, yet. The main reason is because I have never been provided with samples and I have no experience with this medication. I have not written for it yet because, if I am going to give a patient a stimulant for the fatigue associated with fibromyalgia or chronic pain, I want to prescribe a generic medication especially when off-labeling the medication. Generic stimulants are more affordable, not to mention the brand name stimulants, often will require a preauthorization which will be denied by the insurance company, because they are not FDA approved for "fibromyalgia associated fatigue." The insurance company will have no problem with the patient paying full price for the medication (no portion of the cost of the medication will be covered by the health insurance plan). Paying full price for brand name medications will be absolutely cost prohibitive for the vast majority of people. There may be a situation, where a patient may be able to afford an expensive medication for a "one time" medical issue, but unable to afford to pay for an expensive medication on a monthly basis, such as, in the case of managing fibromyalgia and other chronic painful conditions.

Another drug, which deserves honorable mention, is a medication named Strattera (isatomoxetine hydrochloride). This medication is characterized as a Selective Noreinephrine Reuptake Inhibitor. The exact mechanism by which this drug exerts its effect on the brain is unknown, but I will prescribe this medication to patients, with either fibromyalgia or chronic pain, who complain of confusion and an inability to concentrate. This is a medication, which has an FDA indication of treating ADD/ADHD disorder in both the pediatric and adult population. I do have some patients, who take this medication for poor memory and concentration, and it has been quite helpful. It does not have a generic form. Patients with fibromyalgia and chronic painful conditions often experience problems with focusing on a given task. Certainly, there may be many reasons why a patient may have impaired thinking capacity. [Note: I am specifically talking about memory, concentration and focusing disturbances in patients with fibromyalgia and chronic pain issues, who do not have organic brain disease, which could also present with memory, concentration and focusing abnormalities, amongst other things, too.]

Poor memory and concentration in the setting of chronic pain and fibromyalgia can be due to one or more factors. As we now already know, poor quality sleep is a major cause of thinking and concentration disturbances. Stress and anxiety can cause thinking abnormalities, such as, forgetfulness, poor memory, concentration deficits and the inability to carry out simple tasks and follow directions. Medications can have an impact on thinking capacity. I often will write out instructions for the patient and specifically have the patient read back to me what I just handed them. I want to be sure they completely understand the instructions; I always print the instructions so there should be no confusion from my end of things.

The two main reasons I write out the instructions are because, first, I want to make sure the patient knows exactly what I want them to do; and second, I want to avoid a phone call, especially out of office hours, and have to repeat the process. I have so many patients (thousands) and when I get a phone call out of hours, while I am away from the office, it is just about impossible to remember exactly what each patient is taking and their specific regimens. The bottom line is, whenever I am talking over the phone with a patient (while at the office), I need to have their chart in front of me, so I can review my last note to remind myself, what was done at the last visit. This becomes quite a process: to have to pull the chart; document the conversation; and then possibly call in a new script to the pharmacy or have to mail the patient a new script. Try getting three or four of these in a morning or afternoon when you are trying to see, your already scheduled patients; just one of the many reasons doctors run late. Do not get me wrong, I certainly want to take care of my patients, hopefully that can be accomplished during the office visit.

SECTION EIGHT

Narcotics

Introduction

Narcotics (opioids) represent both a very important and a very effective medication for the management of all types of chronic pain. While there are a great many patients out there who suffer from chronic pain who should be on a judicious opioid drug regimen for the management of their chronic pain condition, not all types of pain are appropriate for the use of these medications. It is tough enough for patients to get appropriate pain management for acute painful conditions which are not expected to be chronic conditions, such as, post-operative situations or in cases of broken bones, let alone chronic conditions where there is no hope of a self-healing process. The latter presents a more difficult situation for the patient to get appropriate long-term relief from the healthcare community.

The medical community needs to understand that large segments of our society suffer from painful conditions. Within this segment are members who are appropriate candidates for opioid management. Narcotics are not bad. They are not just for drug dealers and drug addicts. The origins of narcotics have not been the streets, rather, these medications have their roots in hospitals and clinics and this concept has to be recognized and remembered. These are not evil medications. They are good medications. They enhance the quality of life. They make people more functional. They are just as important as medications for diabetes, blood pressure, cholesterol, thyroid and seizure disorders.

Not only do doctors and patients need to understand this concept, but also, the family members and friends of patients, who take narcotics, need to understand the value of these medications. Patients who take narcotics under the supervision of a doctor for the management of chronic pain are not drug addicts! They may certainly be "drug dependent," but the same can be said about a diabetic who is "drug dependent" with insulin; however, they are not addicted to insulin.

I treat many patients with chronic pain. The management of chronic pain is very subjective. Not all chronic pain patients need to have a narcotic as part of their medication regimen, but many do. The goal is to identify the process which is causing the pain and approach the management sensibly and effectively. This sounds easy enough, but in reality it can be quite challenging for the healthcare provider. The patient really is at the mercy of the treating doctor.

I have found, throughout the years, it has been very difficult for patients to receive effective pain management in the primary care setting. Fibromyalgia is a painful and complex condition whereby pain is just one of its components. Diagnosis and management of this condition is extremely problematic.

For the majority of healthcare providers, who do not believe in fibromyalgia, I really think it is because they do not understand the condition. When there is lack of understanding, it is easy to dismiss the issue altogether. Think about it: how can you expect a healthcare provider to treat a condition which they poorly understand; has probably had minimal, if any, formal training in the subject; and up until recently, there had been no FDA approved medications for its treatment? As I have already stated, even the three approved (at this time) medications for the treatment of fibromyalgia (Lyrica, Cymbalta and Savella) are probably not going to be effective as single "initial" agents for the successful management of fibromyalgia (my experience).

It takes a long time to be good at managing fibromyalgia. The healthcare provider has to feel comfortable with making a diagnosis; a decision to treat; and have familiarity with a host of medications, which I have already discussed [Note: This was by no means an exhaustive list.]; and have the confidence to prescribe medications, in an off-labeled fashion. This is quite an order to fill. You really cannot expect your average (or for that matter above average) healthcare provider to have the proficiency for managing fibromyalgia, a condition which really belongs to the rheumatologist. The problem is there are not enough rheumatologists to treat all of these patients and, as I have already mentioned earlier in the book, many rheumatologists do not want to see fibromyalgia and chronic pain patients.

In Tucson, Arizona, where my practice is located, several of the rheumatologists will not see a fibromyalgia patient. If a patient calls the office of one of these rheumatologists and up-front (over the phone) states they have fibromyalgia, the receptionist will tell them the doctor(s) does not treat fibromyalgia and that is the end of that. Unfortunately, sometimes a fibromyalgia patient will get through to the appointment only to be told, at the end of the visit, they have fibromyalgia and have to seek treatment elsewhere.

Not all rheumatologists manage chronic pain. By the time I finished my Fellowship training in Rheumatology at Dartmouth, I hardly treated any patients for chronic pain. These patients were not managed by the Department of Rheumatology. I was used to treating patients with rheumatoid arthritis, lupus, tendonitis, bursitis, and a host of other conditions which did not require ongoing opioid management. When I went into private practice (straight out of Fellowship), I would have patients who were sent to me with chronic pain issues, many of these patients were already on narcotics and were still having significant pain. I would evaluate the patient and then send the referring physician a letter stating they did not have an autoimmune condition, and they should be sent to a chronic pain clinic. This certainly got me off the hook, but the visit really did nothing for the patient. This process went on for years. It is not that I was lazy; I just did not know what to do with these patients. I did not have the experience with narcotic management. It took many years for me to get to where I am today with my knowledge, experience, and comfort level with managing chronic painful conditions. You might say, in many ways, with regard to chronic pain management, I was self-taught.

Patients would come to me after seeing a host of other doctors complaining of their pain and suffering. Little by little I began to write narcotic scripts for these patients. Many of my patients with chronic painful conditions were seeing a pain specialist. They were also seeing me for the management of their connective tissue disorder. It would not be an uncommon scenario for a patient to see me for the management of their rheumatoid arthritis and the pain specialist for the management of their chronic lower back pain. I would communicate with the pain specialist either in writing or by phone. I was a keen observer on how their pain was being managed. I began to see how these patients were improving with their chronic pain conditions because of the treatment from the pain specialist. As time went by, I was able to see, firsthand, patients could be treated effectively with complex pain medication regimens and still be able to function, even better, because of the successful pain management. I became more comfortable with narcotic prescribing because I was able to see these patients were not abusive with these medications, which were effective with changing their lives in a positive way. The elderly could safely take these medications, and I became comfortable knowing I could prescribe pain medications without harming the patient. I do have to give thanks to my colleagues who taught me pain management without knowing it.

It is not exactly that easy to become comfortable and successful with chronic pain management. This is a process that took well over a decade to get to where I am today; it is an ongoing and evolving process. I learn from my patients and colleagues daily. It took me a long time to feel comfortable with prescribing combination narcotics for the appropriate patient. I actually have some patients who need three different narcotics on board to effectively manage their pain. To get to this level of medication prescribing and management is a long journey which has to be taken to get to this destination. The take home message is chronic pain management on the part of the physician is not for the meek. It takes a long time to know what you are doing and to feel comfortable with these types of challenging patients. They are all around you and I suspect, the majority of people who are reading this book have a chronic pain issue, and continue to search for relief.

Narcotics

I do have a bit of an issue, when a patient is sent to me from a local doctor, who has been prescribing narcotics to the patient for several years, and then one day decides they do not want to prescribe these medications to the patient anymore. When they finally get to me; they are usually on the last week of their prescription and are under the impression I am now going to be the one to continue to prescribe their narcotics. I really do not mind assuming narcotic management for "most" patients. I do recognize chronic pain is a real condition, "pain is pain." However, I do have a bit of a problem, when another doctor puts a person on a long-term narcotic regimen when, in my opinion, after meeting with and examining the patient, and reviewing prior medical records, if available, I determine other (non-narcotic) medications should have been used first to address the problem. It is like going from the first floor to the fifth floor without passing through the second, third and fourth floors. I do believe, the referring doctor had good intentions, and there was a slow evolution of treating a symptom and not addressing the primary cause. In many of these situations, the basic problem is, I now have inherited a patient with a narcotic requirement; and in all likelihood need to continue narcotics on an indefinite basis.

As a general rule, in my experience and observations of managing chronic painful conditions for over two decades, patients who have been on long-term narcotic treatment for chronic pain will always have a narcotic requirement. You cannot take backwards steps, when managing these patients, when it comes to narcotic prescribing. However, it may be possible to use other classes of medications to work along with the narcotic(s) to facilitate better pain control, without the need to increase or expand the narcotic regimen.

Sometimes, narcotics are the only option, if this is the case; I would at least like to know what has or has not worked in the past. There is a great deal of responsibility the physician has when prescribing narcotics. Of course, the patient's best interest comes first, but the physician comes in a close second. There are guidelines for narcotic prescribing, which need to be followed for both the safety of the patient and for the doctor; so that the doctor does not jeopardize his/her license to practice medicine. I know of several doctors, who have been sanctioned by the Arizona Board of Medical Examiners with regard to prescribing narcotics, for various reasons. Certainly, for some doctors, it may not have any impact on the running of their medical practice. As you can probably imagine, if your practice is devoted to chronic pain management, and almost every other patient, in your medical practice, is on a narcotic regimen, you cannot afford, for both you and the patient, to lose narcotic prescribing privileges. I will talk more about narcotics and the management of patients who require them a bit further into this chapter.

Moving forward, let us now focus on the use of narcotics in the management of fibromyalgia and chronic painful conditions. As a general rule, the majority of patients with fibromyalgia should not require narcotics for pain management. Most of the time, patients, in my practice with fibromyalgia, who are on narcotics, had them prescribed by another provider. Usually, these patients were fast tracked to the narcotic from their primary care provider; when I take a complete medication history review; it appears my method to the approach of fibromyalgia medication management was not employed; and several classes of potentially helpful non-narcotic medications were bypassed. Unfortunately, for the patient (and now me), the task of pain management now becomes more complex. Already, the patient is taking a narcotic, in a situation where I would not have prescribed it, their pain is not controlled in spite of being on the narcotic, and I have to embark on a somewhat confrontational discussion about it. The bottom line is, patients, who take narcotics for chronic pain are unlikely to come off of them; this is a difficult situation. At the end of the day, I have to work with what presents to my office. Of course, their present pain management regimen may not be what I would have prescribed; but it now becomes part of my ownership. In these situations, it is possible to add another medication which is a non-narcotic to take up some of the slack, but in all likelihood, either I will need to increase the dose of the narcotic; change the narcotic to another narcotic; or possibly add another narcotic to the medication regimen. For the time being, I will just talk about the use of narcotics in patients, who come to me for chronic pain management, who are not already taking a narcotic.

True or false, narcotics are not appropriate for the management of fibromyalgia? The answer (in my book) is false! It is my opinion (and experience) that narcotics are not necessary or appropriate for "most" patients with fibromyalgia. Having said this, there are subsets of patients, who will need a narcotic (an opioid) for the management of their pain. Sometimes, a patient's pain is not adequately controlled, even with combinations of multiple different classes of non-narcotic medications; and the only other medication alternative is an opioid. As you can imagine, this can be quite a problem for a patient, who is appropriate and needs a narcotic for pain management in a condition (such as, fibromyalgia) which many healthcare providers do not even believe exists.

So, who gets the narcotic? Are narcotics just for the middle-aged with chronic pain? Is a narcotic appropriate for an elderly patient, or inappropriate for a young patient? [Note: For the purpose of this book my discussions regarding the use of narcotics will specifically be in reference to the use of these medications for the treatment of fibro-myalgia and other chronic painful conditions.] Who should be treated with a narcotic? The answer is, "Whoever is appropriate for ongoing opioid management."

It is not about the age of the patient. It is about what is necessary and appropriate to treat a painful condition. For example, let us say that a twenty-six year old male comes to my office with chronic right lower extremity pain of three years duration. This person was in good health until he was involved in a motorcycle accident. Several bones of the right lower extremity were broken, multiple surgeries were required, and the patient has been experiencing chronic right leg pain ever since his accident. He has been to multiple doctors: ortho-pedic surgeons, physiatrists, pain specialists and psychiatrists. He has been depressed for several years since the accident. He has been on a host of non-narcotic medications; but unfortunately they have not been successful in alleviating his discomfort.

In addition to his present pain management regimen, he is now given a narcotic, and there has been great improvement with his pain; it is by no means gone, but life is more tolerable and he is able to do more things in comfort. Obviously, this is quite a complex problem for a young person to have to deal with for the rest of his life. The bottom line is, this person's life has changed since the accident, and it is my job to improve this person's quality of life. Here is a situation where this person will probably need to be on a narcotic for the rest of his life. The fact of the matter is this person sustained life altering injuries that are just not going to get better with time; this process of pain has been going on for three years and is not going to get better on its own. The body only has so much capacity to heal from an injury. That is the issue with chronic painful conditions; they are not going to get better by our body's own natural healing process.

The good news is, they can be managed, that is why it is called "chronic pain management," it is not chronic pain "cure." The most likely problem, this patient will encounter with the medical community, is that doctors, who are not chronic pain specialists, may have a problem not only prescribing this patient a narcotic, but with giving this patient the narcotic on a long-term basis. Unfortunately, some doctors will only prescribe a narcotic until they (the doctor) have reached their comfort level of prescribing the medication. I cannot tell you how many times a patient comes to me with a chronic painful condition, who, in my opinion, is appropriately taking a narcotic, sometimes for several years, and the patient tells me their doctor no longer wants to continue to prescribe the narcotic; this really is true! Obviously, this is a pretty bad situation for the patient who, in spite of the long-term narcotic usage, their pain remains poorly controlled. It is a tough situation for the doctor because they have journeyed to an area with the patient, which now extends beyond their comfort level as a treating physician. In the end, both the patient and physician lose out.

Doctors (in general) have a hard time writing for narcotics on a regular basis for young people with chronic pain, this has been my observation throughout the years. My rule for opioid prescribing is I give them to patients where it is appropriate to prescribe them. It is not about the age, I prescribe them where they are needed.

Getting back to the elderly population, who experience chronic pain, I do feel bad for this segment of our population, when it comes to their pain management. An interesting phenomenon about patients in their late 60's, 70's and 80's is that these people are, for the most part, from a generation of non-complainers when it comes to suffering in silence. For this age group of patients many should not be taking NSAIDs for a variety of reasons. Many healthcare providers are afraid to give these patients a narcotic for pain management. There may be concerns a narcotic will suppress the patient's ability to breathe causing them to have respiratory arrest. There may also be the belief an elderly patient will not be able to handle a narcotic; they will be falling all over the place, or will not be able to think clearly, or wake up.

Regardless of what the thinking may be, narcotics are quite safe and effective in the elderly population. I truly believe that of all the medications elderly patients take for various conditions, opioids are one of the safest. Opioids are not associated with an increased risk of ulcers or bleeding. They do not adversely affect kidney function; and many are quite inexpensive. Sometimes, an opioid is the only medication which will be effective for managing chronic and severe pain. There are some situations where I actually have to use combination opioids in the elderly (and younger population) for the management of pain. I will talk more about this as we move further along in this chapter.

Patients, who require opioid management, may have a hard time getting what they need. Many doctors do not feel comfortable writing long-term narcotics, especially when there is subjective pain which is being managed. Most doctors do not have a problem with writing for narcotics in a post-surgical (after surgery) situation or after a trauma. Doctors have more of a problem when writing narcotics for degenerative arthritis, neuropathic pain, and especially, for pain related to fibromyalgia. As already stated, it has been my experience that the majority of patients, who suffer from fibromyalgia, will not require a narcotic for pain management, but some will.

What happens if you are a patient, with fibromyalgia, and you are the one who requires a narcotic for pain control? You are probably going to have a hard time getting treatment unless you see a person, in this case a pain specialist, who understands your problem, and is not afraid to give you what is needed and appropriate, a narcotic for some. Doctors have a fear of regulatory scrutiny. They are afraid of losing their medical licenses. They are afraid of having patients accuse them of turning them into drug addicts. There are probably other reasons which each doctor holds dear to them for not wanting to prescribe a narcotic. This is not a good situation for the patient (and the doctor) when a fear gets in the way of doing what is most appropriate for the patient. When I see a patient, for the first time, who has been living with chronic pain, often for years, what goes through my mind is what will it take to make this person feel good, to give them back their life?

There is a hierarchy (in my book) when it comes to pain management. Narcotics are usually at the top. Some people need to be at the top. There should be a stepwise approach to pain management. The etiology and intensity of the pain will guide me, to my approach with which medications I will use to treat a patient. The past medication history will also be very important. What medications have already been used? Which medications (if any) were helpful? Which medications were not helpful? Which medications worked and then lost their efficacy? What are the other medications on board? Is there another medical condition, which the patient has, which would limit me from prescribing certain medications? Also, I do have to figure out whether the pain is legitimate; is this person a drug seeker? Who sent this patient to me? I always have to beware when a new patient comes to my office and the first thing they say to me is, "I hear that you're the greatest doctor." That usually sends a red flag and I am just waiting to hear the patient ask me for a narcotic.

These are the patients, who neglect to tell me they are taking a narcotic, even when I took a complete medication review 10-15 minutes earlier, but request a specific narcotic refill at the end of the initial visit on their way out of the exam room. I am not saying that all these patients are drug seekers, but it does create an added layer to the problem which needs to be peeled away and figured out. Could this just be a desperate patient, who has gone from doctor to doctor and none of these healthcare providers could get it right? Unfortunately, some patients do manage to fall through the cracks for whatever reason.

Throughout the years I have given lectures to doctors about fibromyalgia and pain management. I have a few favorite questions I like to ask the medical audience before I get started. One question that I ask is, "Do you believe that chronic pain is a real entity?" Another favorite question of mine is, "Do you believe that a person can be experiencing chronic pain in spite of having normal laboratory and radiographic studies?" Finally, another favorite question is, "Do you believe that it is ever appropriate for a patient to require a narcotic on an indefinite basis?" Based on the response to these three questions, I am able to get a sense of the audience attitude, and know how I need to present my information. Obviously, my approach is different when I am talking to general practitioners as opposed to an audience of anesthesiologists and physiatrists (physiatrists are physical medicine specialists, not to be confused with a psychiatrist).

I do not have a hard time prescribing a narcotic to a patient as long as it is appropriate. Every week, I put several new patients on narcotics with the mutual understanding this will be an ongoing requirement for the patient. Narcotics are needed when non-narcotic medications are either inadequate or contraindicated for the management of pain, it is that simple. It took me a long time to develop a level of comfort with prescribing narcotics with the intention of using these medications for ongoing pain management. Also, it is an acquired skill to know when to initiate opioid management. Of course, just because I feel comfortable with writing a narcotic, it does not mean everyone in my practice gets a narcotic. Each patient has to be carefully evaluated, and the decision to write for a narcotic will be made on an individual basis. The ongoing use of an opioid is a serious decision, keeping in mind; the management of any medical condition which involves prescribing medications is serious business. People can get into trouble with any medication which is not used appropriately.

I prescribe many different types of narcotics in my practice for the management of pain. The basic concept to narcotic prescribing is you want to give the patient a medication which is going to be effective for adequate pain control. This is certainly an easy concept to comprehend, but I am amazed to see how many patients are not getting the pain management which is required for various reasons, which I have already discussed. The one which really gets me is when a patient, comes to me, who is taking a narcotic and is still in pain because the dose is not sufficient to alleviate the pain.

There are some basic tenants to writing narcotics for patients. The first one is to give the dose, which is adequate for pain control. As a general rule, the true chronic pain sufferer is only looking for relief. They want the dose of medication which takes care of their pain. It is not good enough for the doctor to just prescribe the pain medication. It takes a short amount of time (a day or two) to know whether a specific dose of a narcotic is going to be adequate for proper pain control. The dosing of the medication has to be geared for the patient's pain control, not to the comfort level of the prescribing doctor. You would be surprised how patients with chronic pain function quite well on either low or high doses of narcotics. One of the biggest fallacies is that patients on narcotics cannot think clearly or function well. One important observation I have made throughout the years is, for the most part, patients who suffer from chronic pain do not function well to begin with because of the chronic pain process. These patients have difficulty with concentrating and following directions. When driving they are distracted by pain or cannot drive well because of limitations from pain; for example, chronic neck pain may interfere with a patient's ability to turn their head.

I have found patients actually function better because of appropriate narcotic usage. They ambulate better; drive better; focus better and remember things better; not to mention that their quality of life is so improved because they are in such less pain. I often have patients who come to me in their 70's, 80's and 90's who suffer from severe arthritis pain. There is no quality to their existence. They have essentially given up on the notion of living comfortably for the rest of their lives. I treat many of these patients with a narcotic (sometimes combinations of narcotics) and they do amazingly well. My philosophy is that nobody, of any age, should have to suffer from day to day with chronic pain. It does not have to be that way.

There are plenty of medications available for the management of chronic painful conditions. The elderly tolerate narcotics quite well. There is no reason to withhold narcotics from the elderly. In fact, I think narcotics are very appropriate for the elderly. They are the most potent medications for pain control. They are compatible with just about every other medication the patient may be taking for other medical conditions. Narcotics are not expensive (some are, but not most). Narcotics are safe to take with blood thinners. Narcotics are not associated with gastrointestinal bleeding, as are NSAIDs. I would much rather treat an elderly patient with a narcotic than an NSAID.

When I determine, it is appropriate to manage a patient with a narcotic, for chronic pain management, I have a very candid conversation with the patient about the nature of long-term narcotic maintenance. There needs to be a mutual understanding that we are moving into the next level of pain management. As a general rule, once a patient requires narcotic treatment for the management of chronic pain they will most likely need to take a narcotic for chronic pain management on a regular basis. This really should be of no surprise to the patient. By the time the patient usually gets to me, they have been suffering for so long, they are happy there is something available for the management of their pain.

Chronic pain management involves entering into a long-term relationship with the pain management physician. There are a lot of "dos and don'ts" the patient has to follow when taking narcotics on a regular basis. There needs to be an understanding that only one doctor should be prescribing narcotics. The patient should no longer receive narcotics from any other physician except the pain management physician. The primary care physicians never object to this since it makes their lives less complicated with regard to writing narcotics, they have enough other issues to deal with regarding the patient's other general medical needs.

When I prescribe narcotics to a patient on a regular basis, there is an understanding they need to keep their scheduled appointments. Narcotic scripts need to be written during the office visit. Patients need to do their blood work as prescribed to monitor various internal organ functions, since medications can potentially affect such organs as the liver and kidneys. I also do in-office urine toxicology screening to verify they are taking the narcotic(s) I am prescribing, and not taking illicit medications, which could create a greater hazard to the patient, who is already taking a prescribed opioid from me. My expectations are reasonable and they are similar to requirements which are outlined by just about any practitioner of chronic pain management. In fact, the Arizona State Board of Medical Examiners (and other State Boards) expects doctors, who prescribe chronic opioids to patients, to adhere to these guidelines. For all of these issues, I have patients sign a Pain Management Contract. This contract is also signed by a witness (one of my office staff members). The patient must adhere to the contract. This protects the patient, as well as me. Breaking the pain contract is the number one reason a patient will be discharged from my medical practice. [Note: It is not just me; be prepared to be discharged from any office if you break a pain contract.]

What constitutes the breaking of a pain contract? Well, there are many things. Doctor shopping for drugs is a major offense. There will be certain exceptions, where I consider it appropriate to receive a narcotic from another doctor while the patient has a pain contract with me. If a person has an accident and is treated in an urgent care or emergency room; a person has a painful dental procedure; or the person has a surgical procedure; these are acceptable reasons for obtaining a narcotic from another physician. It is important for that person to let the other doctor know all the medications they are presently taking. Sometimes another narcotic may be appropriately added to the present medication regimen; and the narcotic, which I am prescribing, may be substituted for a more potent opioid. If a person is getting pain medication from me and then tries to get more or other pain medication from their primary care physician this will create a conflict and breach of contract which will result in the discharge of the patient from my practice. It is not just about my trust in the patient, but also about the potential for life threatening danger, when a patient tries to take more pain medication than they should be taking.

You may wonder how it comes to my attention that a patient is getting narcotics from more than one source. There are many ways in determining this. The in-office tox screen is a pretty good indicator. If they test positive for more substances than I am prescribing (narcotics), that is an easy giveaway. While we are on the topic of drug screening, I always do a baseline in-office urine tox screen, whenever I have a patient sign a pain contract. If the patient signs the pain contract, it is because I am about to put them on a narcotic. It is not unusual for a patient, to come to me for pain management, who is already taking a narcotic from another physician; that is okay. They just have to understand, if they want me to do the pain management, they have to sign my pain contract and abide by the rules of the contract. I tell the patients, they do not have to sign the contract; but if they do not, I will not be able to write a narcotic for them; they will have to either have their primary care doctor do it (a moot point, otherwise, they would not be in my office), or go elsewhere for their pain management.

Throughout the years, I can only think of two instances where a patient refused to sign the pain contract; I never saw them again, go figure!! Sometimes these patients are already on a pain contract from another doctor. In this situation, they can still sign my pain contract with the understanding they cannot get narcotics also from the other doctor. I will also send a letter, to the other doctor, telling them the patient signed a pain contract with me; and I will be assuming the pain management; I have never had an objectionable response to this from another physician.

If I have a concern the patient is getting narcotics from their primary care physician, I will call their doctor to discuss my concern. Another tip-off, that a patient is getting narcotics from more than one source, is that insurance companies have a method of keeping track of all the prescriptions prescribed to their patients from all the patient's doctors. The insurance plans will identify if narcotics are being written by more than one doctor. They will send me a printout sheet, which lists all the patient's medications, their doses, number of tablets prescribed, and the dates on which the prescriptions were filled. I will then have to respond to the insurance company and inform them, of the action, I will be taking to address this issue. I need to document this in the medical record and have a heart-to-heart talk with the patient. Sometimes there is a legitimate reason for what is going on; for example, the patient may have been prescribed a narcotic by their primary care physician a week before initially seeing me. On the surface (according to the insurance company monitoring program) it appears the patient is doctor shopping for narcotics, clearly in this situation this is not the case, end of story. Sometimes, unfortunately, it is the real deal, the patient is trying to scam me, and I have to discharge the patient from my practice.

In the state of Arizona, there is a centralized pharmacy registry system, by which an authorized doctor (like me) can log onto the system by typing in their patient's name and get a list of all controlled medications, that have been filled at various pharmacies throughout the state. This can alert the doctor if the patient is pharmacy and doctor shopping (that is, filling different scripts from different physicians at different pharmacies). Some opioids are quite cheap to purchase with a prescription. A patient could potentially get different opioid scripts from different doctors and fill them at different pharmacies, filling one script using their insurance card, and the other by paying for the medication in cash. This patient could then turn around and sell the medication on the street and make quite a large profit. I actually had a patient pull this scam on me. It took a while for me to figure it out (this patient knew what they were doing). It was a late Friday afternoon, and I was calling two different pharmacies which happened to be out of town, halfway between Tucson and Phoenix, but I was able to verify, that I was being scammed. This took place several years ago, before the centralized pharmacy narcotic monitoring program was up and running. Needless to say, this person is no longer in my practice, and I am that much wiser from the experience.

When I first meet a patient during the initial visit, I need to know up-front, if they are taking any opioids. That is okay if they are; it could be a medication, which is prescribed by another doctor. Sometimes people are taking narcotics they get from friends or other family members for pain management; I do not condone this practice; but I appreciate the patient's honesty. This is actually a good sign to me because it tells me the patient trusts me; and I can begin to trust them. I tell the patient, they need to sign the pain contract if they want narcotic management from me; and they need to give me a sample of urine (now) to perform an immediate in-office urine tox screen. I specifically tell the patient, the tox screen has to match the story I was just told. If the patient tells me they are taking Percocet (regardless of the source), I need to see Percocet show up on the tox screen. If they swear up and down they are not taking any narcotics or illicit drugs and they test positive for an opioid that is pretty much the end of the relationship; I will not be seeing them for a follow-up appointment.

It is imperative for the patient to understand that urine tox screening is very important. As a general rule, historically and presently, I tend to trust my patients, especially the ones I have been treating for a long time. We have a long-term relationship and there is mutual trust. In the past, I did not conduct urine tox screens on my patients. It turns out, at least in Arizona; the Board of Medical Examiners, feels that doctors, who prescribe long-term narcotic medications for their patients have to tox screen the urine to monitor their patients for medication compliance. I know of several, well respected and highly skilled pain management specialists, who have gotten into trouble with the Medical Board for not performing these screening tests. As I began to look around and see what was happening to my colleagues; I came to the conclusion I had better comply with what the Medical Board expects me to do; tox screen the urine of patients, who I prescribe long-term opioids for pain management.

I would send patients to the lab for the urine tox screen. The problem I began to recognize was some patients would take their time about getting the test done. This may have certainly been an innocent process in which the patient did not have the time to get to the lab during the workday. However, there were certain patients, who had no excuse for not being able to do the tox screen in a timely manner.

Besides the lab was only a two minute walk from my office. Specifically, I would tell the patient to go right to the lab after leaving my office. It turned out; some of these patients would get the urine tox screen done, but one or two weeks later. By this time drugs and illicit substances, which would have shown up on a tox screen, the day of the office visit, would be out of their system. In essence the tox screen at that time would be of no value to me.

I needed to figure out a different fail-proof method of tox screening my patients. I then decided to obtain the urine specimen in my office and send it to an outside lab. This was quite a hassle. There was a specific protocol for obtaining the sample. I then had to fill out a lab form; package the urine; and send it UPS to an out-of-state lab. The results would come back a few days later and then I would have to enter the results in the chart. Sometimes the results were confusing or the lab did not test for what I ordered. I would then have to call the lab to discuss the issue with a toxicologist. Interestingly enough, nobody at the outside lab would directly answer the phone; I would have to leave a message for someone to call me back; they would get back to me hours later or the next day. Sometimes, I would get the call-back (on my cell phone) after I left the office; and I would be speaking with the toxicologist without the chart in front of me. I have thousands of patients and need to have the chart in front of me whenever I am corresponding with or about a particular patient. As you could imagine, this was becoming quite an ordeal and time consuming, time I did not have. It was disruptive to the flow of my practice. I had to come up with an alternative method for monitoring these patients.

I decided the best option, for me, to monitor my patients on narcotics was to do the tox screen myself in my own office. This would actually go much smoother from a logistical standpoint, and it gave me control over patients who were deviating from the chain of command by not going immediately to the lab for the test. I was also cutting down on the time it took from sending the urine sample to an outside lab to get a result. It turns out, the cost of the in-office tox screen was less to the insurance company than what they would be paying the outside lab, and it was a win-win situation for everyone in my opinion. This way, I was able to keep consistency across the board. Everyone would have to abide by the same established office tox screening protocol. I only have one problem with this protocol. One insurance company, which will remain nameless, refuses to reimburse me for performing the in-office tox screen (even though I sent them a long letter explaining my rationale for performing the test in my office, not to mention it would cost them less money than if I had to send the sample to an outside lab).

There is a reason why I am telling you about the logistics of narcotic prescribing in my practice; this is not "confessions of a rheumatologist." I want the reader to understand and be prepared for what is expected from a doctor-patient relationship, when it comes to ongoing opioid treatment. If you see a chronic pain specialist, and it is determined that a narcotic is appropriate for your pain management; be prepared to sign a pain contract and abide by the rules. I often have patients question my motive for performing the tox screen. Many will specifically say to me, "Don't you trust me?" with regard to taking their narcotic. I go on to explain to them the reasons for performing the tox screen. I tell them when it comes to narcotic writing, everyone is treated the same, everyone gets tox screened. I will do the urine tox screen every 4-6 months, providing the patient is continuing to take the narcotic. Sometimes, I may need to do it more frequently, if there are inconsistencies between the results of the tox screen and what they should be taking.

It is important to understand each doctor will have a different set of criteria, in which they handle tox screen inconsistencies. For example, I have had patients who have tested positive for cocaine usage. Depending on the patient, for example, how long I have known them, and their prior tox screen history, let us say this was a first time offense, I may deal with this in several different ways. Remember, the reason why I do the tox screen is to verify the patient is taking the narcotic which I am prescribing to them. I also need to make sure they are not taking substances which in combination with what I am prescribing can cause serious problems, the worst being death. In situations where they are found to be taking illicit drugs, such as, cocaine, I explain to the patient, I am not the drug police. I need to make sure they are going to be safe with the medication I am prescribing to them, and they have to understand the combination of their prescription medication and recreational drug(s) use can kill them. I go on to tell them, they need to stop this practice; if they want me to continue to be their doctor and manage their chronic pain. I will tell the patient, I will be tox screening them again (in the near future), and if they test positive again, for that substance or any other substance they should not be taking, I will have no other choice than to discharge them from my practice.

There are, however, situations where I might discharge the patient without giving them a second chance. If this type of issue (a positive tox screen) is identified early on in the opioid relationship; I may just want to quickly end the relationship. I really do not have the time or energy to deal with this type of patient. A word of caution, you really do not want to get discharged from a medical practice because of narcotic noncompliance or illicit drug use or abuse. Remember, this will be well documented in the medical record. It is not uncommon for some doctors wanting to review medical records before accepting a new patient into their medical practice. I like to give patients a chance and the benefit of the doubt. I sometimes get a patient who comes to me with a rather complex set of pain management issues. They have seen multiple primary care physicians and pain specialists. They may have been discharged from another medical practice or two. I want to understand the patient and what the problem was with them and the other doctors. It is not always the patient's fault for a failed relationship with another doctor.

What I need, from the patient, is honesty. I want to know why the patient was discharged. Make sure you are honest with your doctor. Sometimes the patient is misunderstood. It is possible several other prior treating physicians totally missed the boat; and the patient is a victim of the system. This gets back to when I mentioned earlier in the book, it is important for the patient to position themselves with the doctor in a way that the doctor will want to help them. Do not come off with an attitude during the first visit; it will not go well for you. The easiest way for a doctor to distance themselves from the doctor-patient relationship is on the initial visit. There is no established relationship between the doctor and the patient; the doctor has no obligation to treat the patient or see them for any additional visits. Think about it, what happens if you are taking a narcotic and your prior doctor will no longer give you this medication? What if there was an expectation that the new doctor was either going to continue to prescribe this medication to you or put you on something different? You may be in a situation, where you only have two more days of medication before you run out. Then what are you going to do? Repeated trips to the urgent care or emergency room will only help to label you a drug seeker. Think about what you are doing and where you stand with your medication(s) and what you need to do to have a successful relationship with the new doctor.

I sometimes have doubts and concerns with a new patient, with regard to where they stand, with narcotic usage and their true opioid requirement. In these situations; I will have a candid conversation with the patient explaining to them my concern; that I am willing to work with them, with the understanding that I need to get to know them better. I will sometimes say, I do not want to make any changes at that initial visit, and I need to get prior medical records to see what has been done in the past. I will specifically tell them, I expect what they have told me to match up with the records which I will be obtaining from their prior treating physician. Sometimes, I never see the patient again; they just do not come back. On their way out of the initial visit, they just walk out without scheduling a follow-up appointment. [Note: In this situation, they have not signed a release of medical information so I will not be reviewing any medical records.] Sometimes the patient will leave the office telling my receptionist they will call back tomorrow to schedule the follow-up appointment which they never do. Chronic pain specialists know what questions to ask on the initial visit and subsequent visits, too. There are ways of figuring out who is legitimate and who is not. If the patient is inconsistent with their story, this is always a red flag.

Now that we have gotten through the preliminaries, we can begin to talk about specific narcotics I prescribe for the management of chronic pain. Sometimes the narcotic, which I prescribe, is a medication which is added to several other medications, which are on board for pain management; and sometimes the narcotic may be the only medication, I prescribe for pain control. Later on in the book, I will put it all together with various true patient case study examples.

As with other classes of medications, I like to prescribe generic narcotics, when possible. Often they are quite effective for pain management and very affordable. Let us begin with the opioid called Ultram (tramadol). The interesting thing about this medication is, although, it is widely prescribed for pain management by physicians, many are not aware this medication actually is a narcotic. Historically, this medication was non-scheduled (as classified by the FDA), and it is for this reason, many doctors are not aware that tramadol is a narcotic. Ironically, there are presently some states that assign tramadol a class III designation while others still view tramadol as a non-scheduled medication. I will sometimes get a patient who comes to me and tells me their pain is not well controlled on the tramadol their doctor has been prescribing to them. They do not want to take anything stronger for pain, such as, a narcotic. I then have to tell them they are already taking a narcotic, and this creates an awkward situation for me, the patient and ultimately their primary care physician.

One good thing about prescribing tramadol is that a hard copy prescription is not needed to hand into the pharmacy like most narcotics. This means, not only can this medication be called into the pharmacy from the doctor's office, but also refills can be added to the prescription. With most narcotics, the doctor cannot write out refills on the script (technically they can write for refills on the script, but the pharmacy will not issue refills without a new separate script). This medication is available in a 50 mg tablet. The maximal daily dose of tramadol is 400 mg, which can be prescribed as 50 mg 1-2 tablets up to four times a day. There is an extended release form of this medication, which is designed to be administered as a once-a-day tablet, Ultram ER. This medication comes in 100 mg, 200 mg and 300 mg tablets. Depending on your prescription plan coverage, it can be quite expensive. Sometimes, the prescribing physician has discount cards which are provided by the pharmaceutical representative, this can be quite helpful in keeping the cost of the medication down. There is a generic Ultram ER (tramadol ER). However, at this time, it is only available in 100mg and 200mg tablets. Obviously, an advantage of the once-a-day dosing is the medication is delivered in an extended release fashion; there will not be the blood level peaks and valleys that can occur with multiple daily dosing of the immediate release form of the medication. There is no price difference between the generic immediate release and the generic extended release tablets (providing you have a prescription coverage plan; they would both be considered a tier one level medication).

Another similar medication to Ultram (tramadol) is Ultracet. This is essentially tramadol with acetaminophen. Acetaminophen is generic Tylenol. This medication does have a generic form (tramadol/acetaminophen) and is available in a 37.5/325 mg tablet. The 37.5 mg is the tramadol component and the 325 mg is the acetaminophen component. This medication can be written for 1-2 tablets up to four times a day. By having the acetaminophen combined with the tramadol, it allows for less tramadol to be on board. This is an advantage because it allows for a lesser dose of opioid to be used because the acetaminophen takes up some of the work for analgesic (pain) control.

A common opioid, which I prescribe, is Vicodin (hydrocodone). This medication is quite effective for pain management. The active ingredients in Vicodin are hydrocodone and acetaminophen. One advantage, from the doctor's standpoint regarding this opioid is this medication can be called into the pharmacy (a hard copy script is not needed to be brought to the pharmacist from the patient). Also, with Vicodin, refills can be written on the script, so multiple prescriptions are not needed when prescribing this medication to a patient, who is on a stable narcotic regimen. Also, from the standpoint of keeping things "green," Vicodin can be written on a script, which has other medications on it; with many other opioids, the opioid has to be written on its own specific script without other medications written on it. When Vicodin is the only opioid on board, it usually is prescribed 2-4 times a day. Vicodin comes in several strengths which include 5/325 mg, 5/500 mg, 7.5/500 mg, 10/325 mg and 10/500 mg. This is a very effective pain medication when initiating a patient on chronic opioid therapy. This is also a medication which is often prescribed for acute pain management of various conditions.

Another opioid medication, which up until recently, was often prescribed for the management of pain is Darvocet N-100. This medication was withdrawn from the US market in November 2010, but I decided to still mention it in the book because it was on the market for decades and many of the readers may be familiar with this medication. Each tablet of Darvocet N-100 contains 100 mg of propoxyphene napsylate (the opioid component of the drug) and 650 mg of acetaminophen (once again the active ingredient of Tylenol). This medication "was" also available as Darvocet N-50 (50 mg of propoxyphene napsylate and 325 mg of acetaminophen). This medication "was" usually prescribed 1-2 tablets every 4-6 hours, noting the total daily dose of acetaminophen has to be taken into consideration. In general, providing there are no underlying abnormal liver issues, the total daily dose of acetaminophen should not exceed 3000 mg per day. [Note: In 2009 the FDA came out with new Tylenol (acetaminophen) consumption guidelines. They used to say the maximum "safe" daily dose of Tylenol that could be taken was 4,000 mg, now its 3,000 mg. It is important to remember, when taking an opioid which contains acetaminophen, such as, Ultracet, Vicodin, Percocet and formerly Darvocet that one has to take into consideration the concomitant use of acetaminophen (Tylenol).] It should also be noted that beginning in 2014, the FDA has mandated to all pharmaceutical companies that make opioids containing acetaminophen have to limit the acetaminophen component to no greater than 325 mg per tablet. Remember, when using these opioids, in combination with over-the-counter acetaminophen, the total daily dosage of acetaminophen should not exceed 3000 mg per day. There may be certain instances where the total daily dosage of acetaminophen will need to be lower than 3000 mg per day. In some situations, a patient may not be allowed to take any acetaminophen at all, as in the case of patients with severe liver disease.

From the standpoint of the physician, it is convenient to have an opioid, which can be called into the pharmacy over the phone. This is especially helpful for those 4:30 pm Friday afternoon phone calls to the office, with a patient requesting something for pain. There is an added advantage for the patient with regard to having an opioid, which can be phoned into their pharmacy. It allows the patient to go directly to the pharmacy to obtain the medication. If a patient requests an opioid, such as, in the circumstance when an established patient needs something for pain, for just a few days, it saves them a visit to an urgent care or emergency room by having the ability to have a script called into their pharmacy on short notice.

Some opioid scripts can only be filled at the pharmacy. I often have patients, who are on an opioid regimen in which their office visit gets out of sequence, usually because they missed a follow-up appointment for various reasons. Sometimes, they are out of sequence because I had to cancel the appointment. In these situations, the patient usually has two choices. I can write the script for them; and they can come by the office that day to pick it up, or I can put the prescription in the mail; of course, the latter will take several days to get to the patient. Keep in mind, that for the narcotics which cannot be phoned into the pharmacy; they will also not accept a faxed prescription. Remember, if you need a doctor to write you a narcotic script on short notice; do not call 10 minutes before the office is closing. Also, many medical offices may have a 24-48 hour refill policy. Your request for a speedy refill may not occur in the time frame you need it. You will not be very popular with your doctor, if they are getting weekend calls from the answering service to refill a narcotic. I have a no refill on weekend's policy and my patients are all well aware; it is their responsibility to make sure they are not heading into the weekend without enough medication to last them until Monday.

Understand, many doctors have an on-call schedule, and their practice may be covered over the weekend by their partner(s) or by a covering physician outside of their practice. If a covering physician gets a weekend phone call from the answering service stating you need a narcotic refill, in all likelihood, the covering physician will direct you to an urgent care or emergency room facility. Narcotic scams are popular on weekends, especially when another doctor is covering the practice. If you are lucky and the covering doctor is willing to call in a narcotic refill it will only be enough to get you through the weekend. This may create a problem for you, when you try to fill a new script after the weekend; short scripts often proportionally will cost more to fill than a full month supply.

Moving along with my review of narcotics, keep in mind, I will not be talking about every opioid, just the ones I primarily prescribe. The ones I probably will not mention are the ones, which do not have a generic product. There are plenty of generic narcotics around to mention and these are the ones which I usually prescribe.

Percocet, also known as oxycodone with acetaminophen, is a very effective, inexpensive pain reliever. The individual doses of oxycodone and acetaminophen can vary. The most commonly prescribed dose of Percocet is 5/325, the oxycodone component is 5 mg and the acetaminophen component is 325 mg. As with all other medications, which contain acetaminophen (Tylenol), one needs to make sure the daily total consumed dose of acetaminophen does not exceed 3000 mg per day, but also, keep in mind this is providing there is no specific reason the person should have limited acetaminophen exposure, such as, in the case of liver disease. Other doses in which Percocet is available are 2.5/325 mg, 7.5/325 mg, 7.5/500 mg, 10/325 mg and 10/650 mg tablets. Remember, starting in 2014, acetaminophen components will no longer be greater than 325 mg per tablet.

Percocet is a medication which cannot be called into the pharmacy. Also, a pharmacy will not accept a prescription which is received by fax. In order for this medication to be filled by the pharmacy, the patient will need to bring in the prescription. The prescription will not be filled if it has other additional medication requests written on it. Also, the prescription cannot be refilled; even if the doctor writes for refills on the script. The doctor may choose to give you multiple scripts for the Percocet to be filled in succession. In this situation, the date the prescriptions need to be filled must be indicated on the prescription. [Note: As already mentioned, doctors are not allowed to postdate a prescription but they can indicate that the script be filled at a later date.] In this situation the prescription must contain the date that the prescription was written, and the date that it can be filled.

Some pain management specialists will have chronic opioid dependent patients come to the office once a month to pick up the next script. I am not a big fan of doing that. I do think, for most people, this is an excessive practice. To be quite honest with you, if I have to keep such close tabs on a specific patient I am treating with an opioid, chances are I do not want that person in my practice. I am not the narcotic police. I need to dispense narcotics and monitor the patient, in an appropriate fashion. Most of my patients, on narcotic regimens, with whom I have a well-established relationship with, are seen in my office every two to three months. I never give out more than three months of a narcotic at a time. Recently, I have had many patients tell me their insurance company is requiring their doctors write them for a full-year prescription for medications they take on a regular basis (a 90 day script with three refills). Personally, I do not like this practice, even with non-narcotic medications. Certainly, I am not going to do it with an opioid! I tell that to my patients. I go on to tell them, it is more of an inconvenience for me, to have to write more prescriptions throughout the year, but that is fine with me. I do not mind taking the extra effort to do it my way; a 90 day supply with no refills. I believe this is most appropriate for the patient and also myself; I have a medical license to protect.

Percodan is an opioid which contains oxycodone (4.5 mg) and aspirin (325 mg). I really do not write for this medication because chances are, if I have a patient on an opioid, especially in the elderly, I am specifically avoiding any aspirin or NSAID.

One of my favorite opioids, to prescribe, is the fentanyl patch which is the generic form for the brand name Duragesic patch. This is a patch which is worn on the chest wall. The patch is to be worn on either side of the upper chest wall, and a new patch is changed every three days. In some patients, the patch is changed every two days. When the patch is changed the new patch should be placed on the opposite side of the chest. I specifically like to use this medication in the elderly. It can be quite effective for pain management, and it is usually well tolerated. The medication is slowly absorbed through the skin. This allows for a continuous delivery system for the medication. Patients are less likely to have side effects from this opioid, due to less potential for erratic blood levels, as compared to when an oral opioid is taken several times a day. The patch is available in several different doses, which include; 12 mcg/hr., 25 mcg/hr., 50 mcg/hr., 75 mcg/hr. and 100 mcg/hr. The dose is usually started low, between 12 mcg/hr. and 25 mcg/hr. in the elderly. The dosage can always be upwardly adjusted, if necessary.

This medication does come in generic form (fentanyl). There are a few generic brands out there. My experience with the generic versions of this medication is that the Mylan brand seems to adhere to the skin better; your doctor will need to specifically ask for this generic brand, when writing the prescription. You will need a hard copy script for this medication. Ten patches is a one month supply. It might be a good idea to pick up a roll of surgical tape to keep at home, if there happens to be a problem with the patch sticking to the body. It needs to adhere to the body for the medication to be delivered through the skin. There is a specific caution: I tell all my patients, who use this medication, "not" to cut the patch. If you are using a patch and feel the medication is too strong, the patch needs to be removed. Cutting the patch and then placing it back on the skin could potentially result in a drug overdose. The design of the patch is to slowly release the drug through the skin over a 72 hour period. If the patch is cut the medication can be directly and immediately absorbed through the skin, causing an overdose. In fact, before the medication went generic a few years ago, there was actually a recall on some of the patches because of a problem with patches leaking. Also, I tell patients, they should be careful on how they dispose of a used patch. Even though the patch has been used, it is potentially harmful if ingested by a small child or pet. Make sure they are discarded properly.

Sometimes, I have to use combination opioid therapy for the management of chronic pain. The fentanyl patch is a great medication to use as the anchor narcotic, and then add an additional narcotic for breakthrough pain. I can tell you, I often treat elderly patients with combination opioids and the fentanyl patch is usually one of the two opioids that are on board. Patients do quite well, when fentanyl is used in combination with another opioid when it is appropriate for dual opioid management.

Dilaudid, also generically known as hydromorphone, is another opioid, which I often prescribe for pain management. This medication is available in 2 mg and 4 mg tablets. The dosage is started at 2-4 mg, two to three times a day. The dosage can be increased up to 4 mg, two tablets three times a day. Remember, when I talk about drug doses, I am describing what I do in my practice. Under no circumstances should you ever adjust the dose of any medication, which you are taking without consulting with your healthcare provider. Dilaudid is also a medication in which the patient will need a script in hand to get filled; it cannot be called or faxed into the pharmacy.

Another opioid, which has been around for decades is Demerol, generically known as meperidine hydrochloride. This medication is available in tablet and syrup form and by injection if given in an emergency room or urgent care setting. The tablets come in 50 mg and 100 mg strengths. The syrup is available as 50 mg of Demerol per 5 ml. As with all other opioids, the dose is initiated low, usually 50 mg up to four times a day. The maximum dose of Demerol, I will prescribe to a patient is 400 mg per day in divided doses. This medication is not expensive and can be quite effective. As with most other opioids, the script-in-hand rule applies.

Morphine sulfate is another one of those opioids, which have been around for a long period of time. This medication is also quite effective for managing chronic pain and acute pain, too. It is generic, but there are also non-generic morphine products available, one specifically is Avinza, a once-a-day morphine medication. Certainly, there are benefits to a once-a-day opioid, but they do come at a price, they cost more. The drug companies usually have discount cards, which in some circumstances could bring the co-pay down to nearly the same that you would pay for a generic medication or possibly even no co-pay. The trick is you have to be given the discount card from the doctor; however, discount coupons for brand name medications can usually be obtained on-line by going to the product website for that specific medication. I will offer a once-a-day opioid to my patients, but I will explain to them it may be pricey. Even though I know the medication may be expensive, and there may be alternative generics, I always like to inform the patient what is available.

I will sometimes have a patient, who is taking a once or twice-a-day non-generic narcotic, but they may have to change to a less desirable dosing regimen with a different opioid because they have not met their deductible and they do not want to reach it on an expensive medication. They may have to take the alternative medication for several months before they reach their deductible; then I will switch them back to the once-a-day product. Some insurance plans (actually many) have high deductibles, but after that is met there may be a zero co-pay, this may even include medications. Keep in mind, the same insurance company, for example Blue Cross/Blue Shield, will have multiple different plans all over the country, and these different plans may have totally different benefit packages. You should know the benefits of your particular plan. When in doubt just call the customer service number on the back of your insurance card. If you do not feel you are getting the answers you need; just (politely) request to speak with a supervisor. Just be nice along the way and you will get your answers. Do not start off complaining you had to wait 20 minutes just to speak with this person.

Avinza, the once-a-day morphine sulfate, is available in 30 mg, 60 mg, 90 mg and 120 mg tablets. The general rule is to start low and work upwards to the appropriate dose. Remember, when I talk about upwards dose adjusting, this is something for your doctor to do. Do not take it upon yourself to make any changes without discussing it and getting the green light from your doctor. The effects, of an opioid, are quick. It should not take more than a day or two to know how you are responding to a particular opioid. If it is not working after a few days that is as good as it is going to get with that medication at that particular dose. Opioid doses are titrated upwards according to the patient's response and tolerance to the medication. In some ways one can say with opioid dosing, "the sky" is the limit, but not literally. What I mean by this, based on my experience with prescribing opioids to patients for over twenty years, is opioid doses need to be increased to control a patient's pain. Sometimes the dose, which is needed to control the pain, is never reached because of intolerance to the medication; this can be almost anything from an upset stomach, nausea, vomiting, headache, dizziness, light headedness, mental status changes and even allergic reactions. In these situations the medication has to be discontinued and an alternative opioid needs to be considered.

The generic, morphine sulfate is available in an immediate release (IR) form and extended release (ER) form. The ER form is usually prescribed 2-3 times a day and the IR may also be added for breakthrough pain, usually from anywhere from one to four times a day. The idea is to try to have most, if not all, of the dosing to be in the ER form, and just rely on the IR form for rare breakthrough pain management. It may take some time and juggling of the two forms to get the right balance. When I prescribe morphine, I will write for the ER and IR usually together. There is no set rule for dosing. Whenever I write for any opioid, my decision making process will be based on several factors. Has the patient been on an opioid before or is presently taking one? What kind of dosing has been necessary in the past to achieve pain control? Is the patient a "lightweight" when it comes to taking medications in general, that is; do small amounts of medications go far in the patient? Is the patient a heavyweight when it comes to medications, that is; will they need industrial strength doses to ease their discomfort? Just because a person may be overweight does not necessarily mean they will need a high dose of an opioid for pain management. I can think of situations, when I prescribed a relatively low dose of an opioid, to an overweight person; and they could not even function on that small dose of the medication, and other situations where a thin elderly eighty-two year old woman needed a high dose, dual opioid therapy to manage her particular painful condition, go figure! I always tell my patients the dose of opioid needs to be tailored to the individual patient and multiple factors will determine which opioid and what dose will be needed for appropriate pain management.

The doses, of morphine sulfate ER, which I prescribe come in 15 mg, 30 mg and 60 mg denominations. The morphine sulfate IR, which I prescribe comes in 15 mg and 30 mg doses. I actually have a patient, in my practice, who, has a very complex pain process and requires a total of 450 mg of morphine sulfate a day, and this is in addition to methadone, Lyrica, Celexa, an NSAID, trazadone and a few other medications. This is an extreme example of what is sometimes necessary to control pain. This is complex medication prescribing; not many doctors feel comfortable writing these combinations of medications and at high doses. However, there are many people, out there, who require this type of complex medication regimen for pain management. If your average run of the mill chronic pain patient cannot even get simple opioid management from their healthcare provider, what are the severe cases supposed to do? Keep in mind, in no way do I mean to minimize the suffering of any person who is in need of chronic pain management.

Doctors, who practice chronic pain management and feel comfortable with prescribing pain medication, after a while, become quite familiar with the condition of pain. We have an understanding of what patients are going through and what is necessary for treatment. We tend to know when to cut bait, with ineffective therapies and move forward and more aggressively. I will not reinvent the wheel, when a patient comes to see me. Depending on the unsuccessful past medication history, certain contraindications to certain medications, and other medical problems which are present, I will sometimes start a patient on an opioid regimen on the first visit. This is why it is so important for me to spend a significant amount of time on the first visit with the patient to determine, that day in most circumstances, where this patient needs to move forward with a pain management medication regimen.

Often, I have patients, who, come to me with end stage joint disease, such as, a severely degenerative hip or knee. They are taking an NSAID without significant relief and are in need of a joint replacement. For most of these people, they need an opioid for pain control. I tell this to them, up-front, and will prescribe them a narcotic on the first visit. I tell them, in order for them to obtain pain relief they will need the opioid for the time being, until they get their joint replacement. The opioid can always be tapered, after the surgical procedure.

The bottom line is, in this situation (a painful end stage joint); it is unlikely they will experience relief of pain without anything short of an opioid. [Note: It is not uncommon for people, who need joint replacements that have to postpone the procedure for long periods of time, due to a multitude of factors and situations, which range from financial to family and work obligation issues. You cannot expect these people to suffer until they get their surgery. Some patients are not surgical candidates, as they may have other medical problems which preclude them from undergoing a rigorous surgical procedure. In this situation, I tell the patient, I will do my best to manage the pain, usually with one or more opioids. Some patients are physically able to have surgery, but will not opt to have the procedure, preferring to just stick with medical management.]

One last opioid which needs to be mentioned is methadone, the generic form of Dolophine or Methadose. This is a medication, which I often prescribe, for chronic pain management. It is very effective and inexpensive. The dose of methadone will vary from patient to patient, as with all other opioids. When most people hear the word methadone they associate this medication with drug addict recovery programs. When I write for this medication I am prescribing the 10 mg tablet. This can be dosed in some patients as a single once-a-day dose, or in divided doses up to four times a day. I have some patients who take up to 160 mg of methadone a day, with higher doses; the dose is divided throughout the day. This is a medication, which can work well with the fentanyl patch for those patients who may require dual opioid coverage. Here is a situation where very good pain control can be achieved with the combination of generic opioids.

SECTION NINE

Topicals

Finally, there are a few medications, which can be topically administered for the management of pain. There is actually an over-the-counter medication known as capsaicin, the brand name for this medication is Zostrix. This is a medication, which either works or it does not; I guess you can make this statement about any medication! It can be of value for local joint pain. You simply take a small amount (about the size of a pea) and rub it over the painful joint three to four times a day. The way in which this medication works is by depleting something called substance P, a neuropeptide, which plays a role in the transmission of pain impulses to the brain. There are some precautions, which I tell my patients, when it comes to using this medication. Heat, such as, hot water or a heating pad; can activate the medication to cause a burning sensation where it is applied. This will not cause a chemical burn, it will just hurt. It is for this reason I tell my patients to put it on after taking a bath or hot shower or soaking in a hot tub. If this should occur, it can be deactivated by just pouring milk on the area. It works the same way as if you ate chili pepper and your mouth was burning and you drank milk to soothe your mouth. In fact, it is capsaicin, which is in chili pepper and gives it the hot taste. It is for this very reason, I tell patients to make sure they wash their hands after applying the medication because it may cause burning in the eyes and mouth if their fingers touch these regions. It is a very safe medication and inexpensive, if the generic product is purchased.

Another topical medication is Voltaren gel 1% (topical diclofenac). This can be applied to the knee or hand three to four times a day. Its FDA indication is to the knee and hand regions, but I have patients who use it with success on other parts of the body. This medication is actually a topical NSAID. The absorption is about 3%. Theoretically, a person who should not take any aspirin or NSAID may need to even avoid this medication; it will be a judgment call by the prescribing physician. Unfortunately, there is no generic for this medication so it will hit your pocket book or wallet.

There is another topical which comes in a liquid form; Pennsaid, which has the generic name of diclofenac sodium liquid. There is no generic at this time. The FDA indication for this medication is for osteoarthritis of the knee. The dosage is 40 drops which is to be rubbed into the knee 4 times a day. To use this medication on other joints or tendon regions would be an off-label use. It should be noted that for all topical NSAIDs the potential adverse side effects of an NSAID and usage contraindications must be taken into account before using these products.

There are compounding pharmacies which will make various forms of topical NSAIDs. You could go to them and ask what they are able to make. You will need a prescription from your doctor. These pharmacies will, somewhere along the line, have tried to make it known to your doctor they do exist and can prepare these compounds for their patients. Ask your doctor if they are aware of these services which may be provided by a pharmacy near where you work or live.

Honorable mention also has to be made for the Lidoderm 5% patch. This is a non-generic patch, which is applied to a painful region of the body (typically the lower back or knee). This is a prescription medication, whereby, the patch is only worn 12 hours a day. Typically, the patch is applied to the painful region in the morning, after bathing. This patch will not adhere well to the skin, if it gets wet. After 12 hours, the patch is taken off and thrown away. The next patch is then applied 12 hours later, the next morning. Wearing the patch longer than 12 hours is not going to hurt the patient. After 12 hours, the active ingredient of the medication (Lidocaine is a local anesthetic) has dissipated. The response to this medication will vary from patient to patient. Some patients find it very helpful; others claim no value; and some give it mixed reviews. Being a non-generic product, it is not inexpensive. A month supply of this medication will be 30 patches. However, the total daily number of patches that can be prescribed for usage is three. If a person uses three patches a day, a one month script can be written for ninety patches noting that the co-pay will be the same as for the person who only uses one patch per day (30 per month), providing that the prescription is covered by an insurance plan.

Already, I have mentioned the fentanyl (opioid patch). This medication is applied to the skin, gets absorbed into the blood stream and exerts its effect on the central nervous system. There is an NSAID patch called Flector. This is Voltaren (diclofenac) in a 1.3% patch which is changed twice a day. Unlike the Voltaren gel, this patch is designed to work as an NSAID, to help with pain in a systemic fashion as opposed to a local effect. The same precautions regarding all NSAIDs apply to the Flector patch. This medication has only been around for a few years; hence, there is no generic. Just remember, the non-generic medications are usually sampled to your doctor, your first few tubes of Voltaren gel or Flector patches could be for free (samples from your doctor). Ask your doctor if they have any discount cards; they should have them. It does not hurt for you to ask; they may have them and forget to give them to you. It should be noted, medication discount cards do not usually apply to the Medicare population.

Also, sometimes (and this goes for many non-generic medications) the pharmaceutical reps may drop off discount cards directly to your local pharmacy. It does not hurt to ask the pharmacist or pharmacy technician if they have any discount cards behind the counter. While we are on the subject of pharmacist and pharmacy technicians, I would make it a point to be nice to these people. Remember, they are the messengers. They do not make the rules about the cost of your medications or which ones need prior authorization. Sometimes, they will not even be able to give you the price of the medication without actually filling the script first. It is only human nature to not want to go out of your way for someone who is giving you a hard time. Be nice to them; and I am sure they will go out of their way for you. Their job is not easy. They are hearing complaints from people all day and that is not what they are there for. Take your complaint to the insurance company, not the pharmacist. I only mention this to you because it is a reality.

The purpose of this book is to help you along the way with every aspect of what is necessary for you to get what you need for the management of your chronic painful condition. It will be a journey which will involve different health care professionals along the way. This book is your companion and reference guide.

four

Case Studies—Which One Of These

Patients Sounds Like You?

It is now time to put it all together. This is where you should be able to identify with one or several of the real clinical cases which I will be presenting. I actually have pulled select patient charts to present. Although I consider each patient to be unique with their pain issues, many of these patients fall into certain categories, which may mimic what you are experiencing. Remember, this is not a "how-to" book; do not medically manage yourself. Use the information in this book to empower yourself with your healthcare provider. It is not uncommon for two separate patients, presenting with similar symptoms and having the same diagnosis, to be prescribed treatment regimens different as night and day. These cases are presented to illustrate you are not alone in your suffering. There is help out there; providing you get to the right places. Hopefully, by reading the previous chapters, you are moving in the right direction. Remember, I have treated thousands of patients for over 20 years with various painful conditions. Many of these patients may not follow what I call the "typical" pain presentation.

However, I think, by the time you have reviewed these cases, most of you will have identified with at least one of them.

As I was writing this book, I was thinking about the manner in which to present this material. I did not want this to be written like a medical textbook. I came to the conclusion that I needed to take this information directly to the general public; they would know what to do with it. They would be in a position to take this information (with direction and the outline of a proven path to follow) and accomplish something substantial to get the help they need.

The public is much more educated these days. You do not have to be a doctor to learn about medical conditions. The Internet allows you to type in your question and volumes of information are immediately available. The problem, with Internet information, is you have to be careful with what you read. Just because it is in print does not mean it is true and accurate.

I wanted to make sure I could present this subject matter in a way which would be understandable and easy reading. As a doctor, it is important to be a good communicator. I treat patients from all types of socioeconomic and educational backgrounds; I need to be able to communicate with all of my patients; they need to understand what I am telling them; it is my job to make sure this happens.

With each of the following Case Studies, I will start out by providing a brief overview about each patient and discuss pertinent social, historical and clinical information. These overviews should give enough initial information to determine if a particular Case Study sounds similar to conditions you are experiencing. Keep in mind, your issues certainly may differ in some ways from theirs, but the point is to look for generalities between these Case Studies and you.

Case Study Number One:

A forty-two year old white female was referred to my office from an out-of-town neurologist. She last felt well five years ago. Her sleep pattern varied; she did not feel rested in the morning. She fatigues easily; experiences poor memory and concentration capacity. She describes tenderness to touch and irritable bowel, noting she does not have headaches. She was treated with various NSAIDs throughout the years without deriving any relief from these medications. For the past month, she was being treated with Lyrica (150 mg at night). This medication gave her mild relief of her overall diffuse muscle and joint pain.

Her past medical history was significant for two healthy pregnancies (two daughters ages 15 and 20). She had a tubal ligation and tonsillectomy. Family history was unremarkable (with regard to her symptoms). She was not taking any other medications except for the occasional Tylenol (acetaminophen) for headache.

She has been married for 12 years. Her husband is retired military (Army). She was actually born in Germany; has been in the USA for 20 years; and speaks perfect English with a hint of a slight accent. She is a non-smoker and does not drink alcohol. In the past, she enjoyed horseback riding, swimming and dancing.

She informed me her basic blood work was all normal, including her thyroid function. The last time her blood was drawn was about 10 months ago. She presented with no medical records, but she was a very good historian.

Her examination was significant for global muscle tenderness. There was minimal joint tenderness of the hands, without any areas of joint swelling. She did appear fatigued. It was quite pleasant to talk with her.

Analysis:

This lady clearly has fibromyalgia. In fact, the referring physician (the neurologist) had made the diagnosis. However, she was still symptomatic in spite of treatment with Lyrica. One thing which always needs to be ruled out, in anyone who is labeled with fibromyalgia, is hypothyroidism. She told me her thyroid tests were normal; they were done 10 months ago. I certainly had no reason to doubt what she was saying, but I needed to verify her thyroid function was indeed normal. Her set of symptoms could be due to a low thyroid state. As a general rule, a thyroid function test should always be done to rule out hypothyroidism. So, where do we go from here?

The first thing I need to discuss with the patient is I am in agreement with the diagnosis of fibromyalgia. I explained to her, I just want to recheck her thyroid function again along with some other basic blood work (a complete blood count and a comprehensive metabolic panel). I need to have a baseline profile of her blood work just in the event there is an abnormality which could possibly alert me to something else, which could be on going. Also, I like to make sure there are no contraindications for me when it comes to prescribing medication; another reason why I want to see the basic blood profile.

This patient was already taking Lyrica 150 mg at night; she was deriving minimal relief from this medication. [Note: Earlier in the book, I mentioned although Lyrica has an FDA indication for the management of fibromyalgia, it has been my experience this medication does not work well as a single agent for fibromyalgia patients.] This medication is usually prescribed 2-3 times a day in doses up to 600 mg per day for several other FDA approved non-fibromyalgia conditions (the FDA approved total daily dose of Lyrica for the treatment of fibromyalgia is 450 mg, whereas some of my patients only respond well to 600 mg per day; this would be an example of off-labeling a "dose" of a medication).

The fundamental problem with this case is she is not experiencing a normal restorative sleep process. In my experience, Lyrica, when used as a primary therapeutic agent, is not going to correct the sleep process. As a general rule, I want to start off with one medication, when addressing the fibromyalgia patient. I did not feel increasing the Lyrica was going to get her too far. Also, Lyrica is expensive; there is no generic. She was actually getting samples from the neurologist. All things considered, I needed to stop the Lyrica (at least for the time being). In my opinion, there were other ways of addressing this case, including the use of generic medications in an off-labeled fashion. I want to help all of my patients in a cost-effective way without compromising their medical care.

Here is what I did. I first validated the diagnosis. After living with this condition for 5 years, she needed to know what was going on, and more importantly, where she was going. I explained to her there was effective treatment available, and it would not be expensive. I then explained to her the concept of off-labeling medication for the management of fibromyalgia. By the end of the visit, we were on the same page, and a treatment plan was discussed and implemented.

After telling her to stop the Lyrica, I told her I wanted her to begin generic Ambien 10 mg (one tablet) before going to sleep, and I specifically stated this medication should be taken as she is getting into bed. [Note: I had started her on the 10 mg Ambien; this was before the new FDA recommendation of prescribing to women not more than 5 mg of this medication.] I advised her not to eat at least one hour before taking the Ambien, as this will interfere with the effectiveness of Ambien (by causing less absorption of the medication). There must be no alcohol nightcaps with Ambien, as this can be associated with visual hallucinations and increase the potential for sleep walking and doing other activity, after going to bed without memory of the event in the morning. Some people have gotten in their cars and driven places without any recollection of the event. [Note: This is a phenomenon which is not just specific to Ambien; reports of similar behaviors have been associated with other sleep aids, especially when combined with alcohol.] I also sent her for some baseline blood work: a complete blood count; comprehensive metabolic panel which includes liver function; kidney function; and electrolytes. I also sent her for a TSH (thyroid stimulating hormone; a thyroid blood test) and a complete urinalysis. Her follow-up appointment was scheduled for two weeks later.

When she returned two weeks later the report from her was that she was feeling the same, but in addition to this she was having nightmares, clearly from the Ambien. Her examination was without change. Now what?

I stopped the Ambien and started her on Klonopin (clonazepam). The instruction was to take 0.5 mg of Clonazepam, at bedtime, and to increase the dose to two 0.5 mg tablets (at bedtime) in one week, if tolerated and not improved. This medication falls under the class of a benzodiazepine; the same category as Valium. Some doctors may not feel comfortable prescribing this medication on a long-term basis. In this particular situation, I chose to also put her on Neurontin (gabapentin). The use of both of these medications, for the management of fibromyalgia, is off-labeling. I have been successfully prescribing these medications, and others, for years for the management of fibromyalgia. Remember, Neurontin is a medication that has an FDA indication for the management of certain types of seizures. It is actually the parent of Lyrica. This medication comes in a generic form as opposed to Lyrica. The clonazepam was for the sleep disorder and the Neurontin was for the pain (Neurontin is not a narcotic). Neurontin often can help with a poor sleep pattern. The initial dosing of Neurontin (in this situation) was 300 mg three times a day with the last dose to be taken at bedtime, with the clonazepam. I have found taking the last dose of Neurontin at bedtime can be helpful in many patients with sleep problems, in addition to their sleep aid. I needed to see her two weeks later for the follow-up appointment.

At the time of the next visit she was delighted to tell me she was feeling great. She was only using one tablet of clonazepam (0.5 mg at bedtime) and the Neurontin 300 mg three times a day (last dose with the clonazepam). She was sleeping well, experienced a restorative sleep process and her pain had resolved. She felt like a new person. Her family and friends noticed a significant change in her, for the better. She was back to her old self and beginning to enjoy life again. [Note: All of her blood work and urine test returned normal.]

Here is an example of what I consider to be a straightforward case of fibromyalgia. For years she was misunderstood. She responded well to the off-labeling of two generic medications. I have been treating her for a little over five years now. She continues to do well on the present doses of these two medications. Her follow-up appointments are every three months with the understanding to see me sooner if she should develop any new fibromyalgia related problems.

I will admit this was an easy case to manage. I guess I was lucky with the combination of these medications doing such a great job for her in just a short period of time. With all honesty, she is more the exception to the rule with regard to her doing so well so quickly. The cases do get tougher as we forge ahead. Does she sound like you or anyone you know?

Case Study Number Two:

A seventy-six year old widower (referred to me by his significant other who is also a patient of mine) presented with the complaint of disabling lower back pain along with neck pain, but to a significantly lesser degree. He has a history of prior neck and lower back surgeries. The pain in the lower back is so severe he cannot lay flat when he goes to bed at night; he has to sleep in a recliner.

His past medical history is significant for depression, heart beat irregularities (arrhythmia), gastroesophageal reflux, right shoulder joint replacement and peripheral neuropathy.

His present medication regimen consists of Neurontin 300 mg three times a day (for his peripheral neuropathy); Wellbutrin 150 mg twice a day (an antidepressant); metoprolol 25 mg one tablet a day (for the abnormal heart rate); Celexa 40 mg one tablet each morning for his depression; several vitamins; a daily baby aspirin (81 mg), and for his back and neck pain Percocet 5/325 one tablet up to three times a day and methadone 10 mg twice a day. He also takes 20 mg of Prilosec each morning for his reflux.

Blood work results, which I requested from his primary care physician's medical records, revealed an elevated creatinine (one of the measurements of kidney function) indicating renal insufficiency. His complete blood count was normal.

Examination revealed an elderly white male who was clearly uncomfortable. He was alert and oriented and responded to all questions appropriately. There was limited neck range of motion and tenderness. His lower back was very tender to touch. He ambulated slowly with a chair walker.

Analysis:

This is a perfect example of an elderly patient who presents with chronic pain from degenerative joint disease. It is quite evident that he has significant neck and back issues. He really has no quality of life.

In spite of the fact he is taking two opioids (Percocet and methadone) he is still miserable. This is unacceptable management. He should be experiencing much less discomfort than what he has been dealing with. Remember pain management is relative. The concept with pain management is, the patient is never too old (or young) for treatment. We need to identify the etiology (cause and origin) of the pain. In this case it is a no-brainer, we know his problem. We now can immediately proceed to "what to do about it."

The first thing I have to think about is what will be safe for him to take. I need to consider his advanced age, along with some of his other medical issues, when determining which medications will be the most appropriate to manage his chronic pain. He has a history of kidney insufficiency; medications which can potentially interfere with kidney function should be avoided (such as NSAIDs). Because of his age, I prefer to "not" use an NSAID for many reasons. He has a heart condition, and the incidence of congestive heart failure is 13 fold greater when an NSAID is used in these patients. I also want to spare his kidneys from the potential negative effects from this class of medication. He has a history of gastric reflux for which he is taking Prilosec; adding an NSAID in this situation could increase the risk of gastrointestinal bleeding. Aside from these major issues, I would not prescribe an NSAID to this patient because I can assure you, whichever NSAID would be prescribed; it is not going to be strong enough to address his pain. Keep in mind; opioids are much more potent analgesics (pain controllers) than NSAIDs. He is already taking two opioids and still having pain issues. It makes no sense to consider the use of an NSAID in this patient. The answer to this gentleman's pain problem will be with the use of opioids, but a different regimen than what he is taking. What he is presently taking is not working. The next decision process is to determine, if I want to change the opioids, or modify the doses, or a combination of the two. This is where opioid management experience comes into play.

I had to have a candid discussion with the patient. Clearly, he was not a drug seeker; he was only seeking relief. I told him there was no doubt in my mind I could help him; I have seen and treated this problem hundreds of times before. I saw no reason why he could not have similar success with an appropriate medication regimen. There needed to be mutual understanding that my role was to alleviate pain. I would not be able to correct the problem; however, I could manage his pain with the intention of improving his quality of life.

There were some housekeeping issues which needed to be addressed before proceeding forward. I explained to him, only one doctor should be prescribing opioids. He wanted me to assume his opioid management. I explained to him, he would need to read and sign my three page pain management contract. Finally, I told him, whenever I initiate opioid therapy, I perform an in-office urine tox screen. He signed the contract and submitted a urine sample; the results were consistent with the two opioids which he was prescribed by his primary care physician.

A tox screen is also done on a random basis throughout the course of opioid management. I tell all my opioid treatment patients, everyone is treated the same with regard to the pain contract and tox screening. If, the patient is not willing to abide by the rules of the pain contract, I tell them I will treat them, but not with the use of an opioid, which is another way of me telling them I cannot help them without the use of an opioid. Clearly, if a patient needs an opioid they need an opioid. There is no discrimination with regard to who gets a tox screen. I treat all types of people from all different academic and socioeconomic backgrounds. I treat many doctors who have chronic pain issues; they too sign the contract; need to keep their scheduled follow-up appointments; and do the tox screens, as required by the pain contract.

The prescribing of an opioid is very subjective; the choice of opioid(s) and dose(s) prescribed to the patient will depend on the prescriber's preference and experience in treating patients with these medications. We (as doctors) dispense what we feel comfortable writing; this comfort level develops over time with progressive clinical experience and patient success stories.

It was my decision to discontinue the Percocet. I felt he would do well with a long acting opioid along with another opioid (the methadone which he was already taking) for breakthrough pain. Remember, when appropriately administered and monitored, opioids are very effective for pain management in elderly patients. It is important when seeking chronic pain management that you establish yourself with a doctor, who is very experienced with opioid management, and does not have biases which could interfere with optimum pain management. I started this patient on the fentanyl patch 12 mcg/hr. (the patch is to be applied to the chest wall and changed every three days). I also told him he should continue to use the methadone 10 mg one tablet up to two times a day for breakthrough pain, if needed. I sent his doctor a letter informing him about the new management plan, and that I would be assuming the opioid prescribing and pain management component of his medical condition. I have yet to have an objection from a primary care physician when I inform them I am assuming responsibility for pain management. The plan was to see the patient in two weeks for a follow-up appointment. He was instructed not to cut the patch for any reason as this could cause immediate release of what should be a timed release of the medication, which could cause an overdose. I told him to call me, if any problems should develop before his next visit.

Two weeks later the patient returned. He was doing better, about 50%, which is pretty good for a first visit intervention. There were no side effects from the medication combination, which is an important factor for successful opioid management. I knew we could do better. I then increased his fentanyl dose to the 25 mcg/hr. patch with the instruction to return to the office in two weeks for another follow-up appointment.

At this next appointment, he reported he was doing even better. The medications were well tolerated, and he was actually sleeping in his bed. He was quite pleased with his progress. He continues to do well, enjoys life, and is able to enjoy the company of his significant other.

The important lesson, in this case, is, elderly patients can do quite well with dual opioid management in addressing chronic pain issues.

Case Study Number Three:

A sixty-three year old white female presented to my office with the complaint of right-sided neck pain with associated numbness going down the right upper extremity. This has been a process which began about 8 months ago, and has been progressive to the extent that her symptoms are now constant. Otherwise, she is quite well for her age. She has used several NSAIDs without significant improvement. The pain has interfered with her sleep pattern, and she also has been quite fatigued. Aside from taking Premarin (a female estrogen hormone) she takes no other medication except for Tylenol 500 mg two tablets three to four times a day for her pain. [Note: She was taking this dose of Tylenol (4,000 mg per day) before the new FDA 3,000 mg per day guideline maximum.] She stated the Tylenol was just as effective as several of the NSAIDs which she has taken in the past, noting it did not upset her stomach.

Examination was significant for right-sided neck tenderness, right-upper back musculature tenderness, and some weakness in her right hand grip strength compared to the left. [Note: She is right-hand dominant, right-handed.] Raising her right upper extremity greater than 130 degrees exacerbated her right-sided neck discomfort.

It should be noted, she had already seen a neurosurgeon who had sent her for an MRI of her neck. Interestingly enough, the MRI revealed degenerative arthritic changes at various levels of her cervical spine, several disk bulges, and upper cervical vertebral spinal stenosis (narrowing of the spinal canal where the spinal cord traverses). Her blood work was normal. The neurosurgeon had sent her for physical therapy (2 months ago); this was not helpful, and only exacerbated her symptoms. He saw her in follow-up a week before seeing me, and told her, the problem was not surgical, hence, her reason for coming to see me.

I explained to her, I was not in agreement with the neurosurgeon, and she did indeed need surgery; as you can imagine, this only added to her frustration. I told her, I could help her with her pain (an opioid being the most appropriate medication in this situation for pain management), but this would be like putting a Band-Aid over a cut which needed suturing. This also created a bit of a diplomatic problem for me because I knew the surgeon; I needed to exercise extreme tact in telling this patient, she needed to go elsewhere, while at the same time not trashing the neurosurgeon (that would be unprofessional on my part). On the other hand, my primary loyalty is to the patient, the person who is suffering with the medical problem. [Note: I am quite candid with patients when I am in these situations.] It is necessary to navigate the patient in the right direction; whether it is me or someone else who needs to participate in the management of the medical problem. If the problem is surgical, I have to refer the patient to a surgeon.

She declined the offer of the opioid. I told her, if she wanted to go the opioid route, it hopefully would be a temporary measure until she could get the surgery, which I felt was necessary. This was the dilemma: the surgeon told her, she did not have a surgical problem and I (the non-surgeon) told her she needed surgery.

I gave her the name of another neurosurgeon, and sent him a letter regarding the patient's problem. This is what is known in the medical field as a "second opinion consultation." I told the patient I would like to see her in a month for a follow-up appointment; my intention still was to offer her pain management, if desired at that time. Two weeks later, I received a copy of the hospital operative report; she had the surgery, which technically went well. She saw me in the office two weeks after her surgery. She reported that she was doing great; her symptoms were almost resolved; and there were no post-surgical complications. I will be seeing her on an as-needed basis.

Analysis:

Neck pain is a very common problem, which patients of all ages may experience. As we get older there is no escape from the fact we will all develop some form of degenerative arthritis. People often will have radiographic evidence of degenerative changes even without clinical symptoms. There are several take-home messages from this case. It is not uncommon for specialists, within the same field of expertise, to have different opinions regarding the same patient (clearly the situation in this case example). Sometimes surgery is the only answer to a medical problem. The results may certainly vary from patient to patient, noting there is also the factor of the surgeon's skill. Sometimes there may be an issue which precludes a surgical intervention, but not in this case. Opioids are a good avenue for pain management to bridge the period leading up to the surgical intervention; however, she did not want to take this option. Perhaps, she may have opted for an opioid if she did not have the surgery in such a timely fashion after seeing me. As observed in this case, the patient needed to get a second opinion, from a neurosurgeon, as this would be the doctor who could perform the surgery.

Sometimes you may see a doctor whose best offering is to redirect you to the right path on which you should be traveling. This is what I did by sending her to see another neurosurgeon. This case is also an example of poor management on the part of the initial neurosurgeon. He had the radiographic information, along with a patient history and clinical findings, consistent with a patient who truly needed a surgical intervention. When you have a situation, such as this case, with ongoing progressive pain and focal neurologic features; something aggressive needs to be done. In my opinion, given all the information available to the neurosurgeon regarding this patient, the referral to physical therapy was a waste of time, and there was no real definitive follow-up plan on the part of the neurosurgeon to correct this problem. I also need to mention, I have known the initial neurosurgeon for many years, and I consider him to be a very good surgeon. He has operated on several of my patients, and has done a very good job for them. Sometimes, we as doctors just do not get it right; there can be many reasons for this. We too can have a bad day, but unfortunately the consequences for the patient are significant. Just keep in mind as the patient; it is not an unreasonable request by you to ask the doctor to give you an outline with a time-frame as to the approach and expectations regarding the management of your condition. You should ask, "What if this happens?" or "What if this does not happen?" and "What is the expected time-frame for these things to either occur or not occur?"

From my standpoint, in this situation, the patient was quite pleased with me even though I did not do anything more than refer her to another physician. My job was easy; that is the way it goes sometimes. This case turned out to have a happy ending.

Case Study Number Four:

A fifty-one year old white male with a history of psoriatic arthritis recently moved to Tucson from the east coast. He has a long history of chronic pain. He takes several medications for the management of his psoriatic arthritis, which is under good control. There is also a history of anxiety, for which he takes Xanax, 1 mg three times a day. He has been taking this medication for 8 years. For the management of his chronic pain, he takes Oxycontin 80 mg three times a day (he has been on opioids for 6 years) and for the past three years he has also been using the fentanyl patch 100 mcg/hr. every three days. There has been no change in his medication regimen for several years. He does experience increased generalized pain if he misses a dose of Oxycontin, or if he changes the fentanyl patch a day later than the due date. In healthier days, he served in the Air Force for twenty years and then law enforcement until being medically disabled, five years ago. He is married and has three healthy adult children. After contacting several other rheumatology offices in town, where he was told he would have to go elsewhere because they do not do pain management (they would not write prescriptions for his narcotics), he came to me.

On examination, he appeared quite comfortable. He was alert and oriented and responded to all questions appropriately. He had mild psoriatic skin lesions on his scalp, elbows and knees. There was no evidence of active arthritis. His examination was relatively benign.

Analysis:

This is a good example of a patient with chronic pain who is actually doing quite well on a complex opioid regimen. [Note: I did not mention the other medications, which he is taking for his psoriatic arthritis.] Apparently, he had already been through the task of obtaining adequate pain management. The biggest immediate issue, for him, was finding another physician who would take on his case and continue to prescribe the medications, which he needed. He did bring medical records with him and the records supported his story. He was well acquainted with the concept of the pain contract along with regular scheduled office visits and urine tox screening. He was a straight shooter; I knew what he needed; and I was going to continue his medication regimen. Here are some major hurdles which people in this situation have to confront. He needed two types of doctors; ideally they would be the same person. He needed a rheumatologist to manage his psoriatic arthritis and a pain specialist who would manage his opioids. There are many rheumatologists who will not do pain management; they refer them to pain management specialists. I can assure you, a pain management specialist will not be treating his psoriatic arthritis. His best bet was to find a rheumatologist who also does pain management, me. It is certainly more convenient for him to have a doctor who does both.

As a patient with chronic pain issues, especially if you are well managed and planning on moving away from your established community, you need to carefully plan your move with regard to your treating physicians and prescription refills. When I have patients, who are moving to another city or state, there are several issues which I bring to their attention; it is always very helpful regarding their transitional care. With regard to my chronic pain patients, especially my fibromyalgia patients, I tell them to do some research regarding doctors, who will be in their new area. I always tell them to see a rheumatologist, hopefully one who will do things more or less the way I have been doing things for them. Perhaps, they have friends or family in the area they are moving to, who may have had experience with one of the local rheumatologists, and they could get a recommendation on whom to see or "not" see. If you are doing this blindly, you could go on-line and plug in the city or county and look for a listing of rheumatologists. Local county medical societies can be helpful with furnishing you a list of rheumatologists (or any other type of physician). The American College of Rheumatology has a website which can be accessed, whereby you could look up rheumatologists, by last name or state categories.

Once you have found a few potential rheumatologists, I suggest you call their office and ask several specific questions. You need to find out, if they are taking new patients, as most are. You also need to find out, if they treat your condition (saying specifically fibromyalgia or chronic pain, depending which one you have, you could have both). It is also important to find out, if the doctor will prescribe opioids, especially if you are already taking them. The office staff should be able to readily give you this information. Sometimes you may run into the problem, where a specialist will not see you unless you were referred by a local primary care physician. Then you have the problem of first establishing yourself with a primary care physician. The fact, you are taking narcotics will complicate that process. It is much easier to get a new primary care physician, when you can walk into the new doctor's office and tell that person, you have chronic pain issues, but they are managed by a pain specialist, you have a pain contract, and most importantly, "you will not be asking them to write any narcotics for you." You just want the primary care physician to take care of your "non-pain" medical issues. This introduction by you, to the new physician, will open many more doors for you, trust me on this one!

I always suggest to the patients who are leaving my practice because of moving, they should schedule a new appointment with the new doctor a few months before leaving Arizona. You want to get on the appointment book in a non-urgent situation. You really need to be proactive regarding continued pain management long before you make your move. If you wait to make an appointment until after your move, you may have to wait 3-4 months for the first available new patient appointment. Also, if you find out the name and address of the new doctor, you could give it to your present rheumatologist and have them send a letter of introduction, as this will be quite helpful. It is important to have your medical records with you as you depart for your new home.

Whenever I get a new patient, and there is the expectation I will be assuming narcotic management, I want to see old records. I embrace the diplomatic concept of former United States President Ronald Reagan "trust with verification." Finally, I always want to see my patients, who are moving away, one last time before they leave, one to two weeks before the move. This gives me an opportunity to tie up any loose ends. I will give patients copies of their medical record, and most importantly enough scripts to see them through until they can establish themselves with a new rheumatologist. The number, of scripts I give them, will depend on whether they have an appointment to see a new rheumatologist or not. If they have not made arrangements, I will give them scripts which will last them for three months. I explain to patients, I am only able to prescribe medications to them for only so long after they have left the practice. Also, I have to be careful with the out-of-state writing of narcotics. I tell the patients to have the new pharmacist call me if there are any problems with filling the scripts until they are able to establish themselves with a new rheumatologist. Sometimes the patient is able to establish themselves with a new primary care physician before they are able to see the rheumatologist. The new primary care physician may be uncomfortable with writing the narcotics until they see the pain specialist. Sometimes a phone conversation between the new doctor and me will make the transition for the patient easier, and the new doctor may feel more comfortable in writing for the pain medication knowing that continued long-term management will be facilitated by the new rheumatologist once, this relationship has been established.

There is a lot of good information, I have just given you. This case was not so much about this patient's medical condition, but how to prepare for a move with regard to ongoing management of your medical condition. This information also works for all of your other medical needs. Good luck with your move!

Case Study Number Five:

A sixty-three year old white female with an 8 year history of insulin dependent diabetes was referred to me, for the evaluation of chronic bilateral lower extremity burning pain, of three years duration. She was worked up for peripheral vascular disease noting the lower extremity blood flow studies were normal. There was no associated lower back pain. She had been treated with multiple NSAIDs without significant improvement. The pain was worse at night. Her primary care physician recently put her on Vicodin 5/500 mg (one tablet three times a day), and this was helpful for the pain, but she experienced constipation; this was relieved with a laxative. Her primary care physician did not feel comfortable continuing to prescribe the Vicodin, thus, the referral to me.

Examination revealed a middle-aged white female who actually appeared quite comfortable. Her examination was overall benign. There was no tenderness over the lower extremities. There was no joint swelling of the lower extremities nor was there any lower extremity edema (no fluid retention in the legs). She was alert and oriented and responded to all questions appropriately.

Analysis:

What is her problem? When a person presents with pain and burning in the legs; there are several conditions to consider. Poor arterial flow could cause these symptoms. Clinically, these patients will display signs of poor peripheral circulation, such as, the legs feeling cool to touch, loss of hair follicles over the distal region of the legs, absence of the pedal (foot) pulse and the legs may look bluish and dusky. These features tend to be exacerbated with walking and improve with rest. The vascular studies, which were done via the primary care physician, were reported to be normal. Another thing to consider would be a condition called spinal stenosis. This is when the spinal canal, over a long period of time, becomes narrow, which impinges on the spinal cord and can cause symptoms of pain, weakness, numbness and burning in the legs. [Note: The process of spinal stenosis can occur at any level of the spinal cord.] If the person is experiencing pain and burning in the legs and the reason is from spinal stenosis, the region of stenosis in the spine will likely be in the L4-L5/L5-S1 region. This diagnosis can be identified by an MRI of the lower spine (a lumbar MRI). A clinical feature of spinal stenosis is that the patient will have an exacerbation of their symptoms with walking and they will improve with rest. This is similar to what patients with peripheral vascular disease experience, noting the major difference is that with spinal stenosis, the legs do not feel cold nor turn a dusky color, especially when walking. The medical term for this discomfort in the legs which occurs with walking is caused claudication. There are two types of claudication: vascular (poor blood flow) and neurogenic (the nerve is compressed). The treatments for each of these conditions are different. Neurogenic claudication from spinal stenosis usually responds quite nicely to surgery. Vascular claudication usually needs to be addressed with medication or possibly a surgical procedure to open up the arterial blood vessel diameter to increase blood flow; this procedure is called an arterial angioplasty. Sometimes a graft has to be connected to bypass a severely clogged artery to restore proper blood flow to the deficient region, or the placement of an arterial stent may suffice to maintain adequate circulation.

This patient had neither of these conditions. It turns out that an EMG/NCS (an electrical diagnostic study) of the lower extremities revealed peripheral neuropathy (nerve injury). There are many reasons why nerve tissue can be damaged. In this particular patient, the neuropathy was likely secondary to her diabetes. Fundamentally, the best approach to inhibit the progression of diabetic neuropathy is to achieve and maintain good diabetic control. The issue is that she is symptomatic with regard to her neuropathy, and now she is on an opioid and feels better. The referring primary care physician does not want to continue to prescribe the opioid; the patient wants to continue to feel good, and there is this new expectation where I will be the one to continue to prescribe the opioid. What now?

I could refer the patient back to the primary care physician stating, I agree with the treatment and they are just as adept in prescribing

Vicodin as me. That would have been a cop-out on my part, but most importantly, I did not think the opioid was an appropriate medication for her to be taking, at that point in time. I realized she felt better and tolerated the Vicodin, but I would not have jumped on the opioid band wagon so soon. The referring physician bypassed several classes of medications which may have been quite effective in addressing her pain in a non-opioid fashion. This patient was certainly not drug-seeking; she just wanted continued pain relief.

This case is representative of several issues, which are worthy of discussion. Every now and then, I get a patient referred to me; who is on a opioid; feels good because of it; but should have been treated (in my opinion) with a different class of medication. Personally, I would not have initially treated her with Vicodin. She is experiencing neuropathic pain. There is no inflammation going on here; an NSAID is probably not going to be effective. We already know she has tried several different NSAIDs, without improvement. My experience with treating neuropathic pain is that NSAIDs do not have the capacity as an analgesic to effectively address this type of pain. Also, neuropathic pain will need chronic medication management. As a general rule, I like to avoid chronic NSAID usage in non-inflammatory pain conditions. By now we (you) are aware of the long-term (and potentially short-term) complications of NSAIDs.

As I already have outlined, the various medications in the preceding chapters, my preference of initial medication treatment, in this patient, would have been to go with one of the anti-seizure medications (Neurontin, Lyrica, Topamax, or Lamictal). These medications are often very effective for neuropathic pain management. Remember, Neurontin, Topamax, and Lamictal are available generically. Many diabetics are overweight, and one of the potential side effects of Topamax treatment is weight loss. Topamax seems like the logical first drug to use.

I now had to get into the conversation, with this patient, about telling her I did not feel she should be on Vicodin. I then had to navigate tactfully through the wave of transition from an opioid to a non-opioid, and to do it in such a way, without making it look like the referring doctor made the wrong decision. Consultants, as I am, depend on referrals from the primary care physicians (do not bite the hand that feeds you).

She was quite agreeable to go along with a medication change. I decided to start her on Topamax 25 mg one tablet, twice a day, with the instruction to increase the medication to two tablets twice a day, in one week, if tolerated and not improved. Two weeks later, she returned to the office for a follow-up appointment. She informed me, she was doing alright (the Topamax dose being 25 mg two tablets (50 mg) twice a day), but not as well as when she took the Vicodin (75 % improved, as compared to when she was taking the Vicodin). The Topamax was well tolerated. There was no change in her weight as compared to the last visit. I told her to increase the Topamax to 75 mg twice a day along with the instruction to increase the dose to 100 mg twice a day in one week, if tolerated and not improved. She was seen two weeks later for a follow-up appointment. She informed me, she was doing quite well, as good as when she used the Vicodin. [Note: It was not necessary for her to increase the dose of Topamax to more than 75 mg twice a day.]

In reviewing this case, we have learned a few things about neuropathic pain evaluation and management. Know what you are treating. Use the most appropriate medications for pain control. Pain management can be effectively managed in many circumstances, without the use of an opioid. Know the limitations when employing the use of an NSAID. Finally, think about hitting more than one bird with one stone. In this case, I anticipated the Topamax to be effective for pain control with the potential weight loss as a side effect from the Topamax, as an extra bonus. It turned out after a few months of treatment, a follow-up appointment revealed a 22 pound, unintentional weight loss (from the Topamax). Both the patient and physician (yours truly) were quite pleased.

Case Study Number Six:

A fifty-eight year old white female came to my office for the evaluation and management of bilateral lower extremity pain of three years duration. She was not sent to me by her primary care physician; one of her friends, was a patient of mine. She had several other medical conditions, which were well under control, including: high cholesterol, low thyroid, and osteopenia (low bone mass but not osteoporosis) and a few other minor issues. Her primary care physician had prescribed several different NSAIDs, which were not helpful. There were no specific studies that were done except for basic blood work, which revealed a normal complete blood count, normal comprehensive metabolic panel and normal thyroid studies (she was getting adequate thyroid replacement on her present dose of Levothyroxine). Other medications included Zocor for her high cholesterol and alendronate (generic Fosamax) for her osteopenia. She also took several over-the-counter products, which included calcium, vitamin D, a multivitamin and 81 mg of aspirin.

Her examination was significant for a right arm sitting blood pressure of 140/90 (elevated), a soft heart murmur, which had been present for years, clear lungs, no muscle or joint tenderness and no joint swelling. There was, however, swelling in her legs, which extended to just below the knees. It should be noted, the time of her office visit, with me, was 10:15 AM. After examining her, I proceeded to ask her a few more questions. I asked her if at the end of the day, were her legs even more swollen? The answer was, "Yes." Was the pain in the legs worse as the day progressed? The answer was, "Yes." Did the swelling improve in the morning, when she got out of bed? She responded by telling me, the swelling was gone in the morning. The last question I asked was; how many times at night did she get up to urinate? She said, "Twice."

I advised her to continue with her present medication regimen. However, I did prescribe a diuretic (Dyazide 37.5/25 mg) to be taken in the morning. I wanted to see her in a week.

When she returned a week later, she told me her legs were feeling much better. Her blood pressure was down to 110/70 in the right arm sitting position and there was no evidence of edema (swelling in the legs). [Note: The time of this appointment was 4:00 PM. When asked how many times she was getting up to urinate at night she told me "none;" a quick fix to a chronic problem.

Analysis:

This is a very common problem, which presents to my office; painful legs. This case is different from the preceding case. It was quite evident to me that her problem, pain in her legs, was secondary to fluid retention. As people get older (not that fifty-eight is old), they have a tendency to retain fluid. There can be many reasons for fluid retention; poor circulation, certain medications can be associated with fluid retention, dietary factors, such as, a high salt intake, heart and liver disease and several other factors. In this case, she had what is called "dependent edema." As the day progressed, while in the upright position, she was retaining more and more fluid. This process of fluid retention can be quite painful. It can also be quite fatiguing because fluid retention is like walking around with water bottles strapped to your legs. Several pounds of fluid can accumulate in the legs by the end of the day. When the patient went to bed, the circulatory system was not working as hard against the force of gravity, when lying down as compared to standing up. What was happening, while she was lying down in bed, throughout the night was that the fluid (edema) began to get reabsorbed back into circulation. The reabsorbed (extra fluid) then circulates through the kidneys where urine is produced. Since the body does not need this extra reabsorbed fluid which is being filtered through the kidneys, large amounts of urine are produced and delivered to the bladder. The bladder can only store so much urine before it needs to make way for the newly brewing supply. She was waking up several times at night, to relieve her bladder. When she woke up in the morning the edema was gone. Then the process of re-accumulation of fluid would start all over again and the cycle continues.

I gave her the diuretic to address the fluid retention. The concept was to make sure she did not accumulate fluid throughout the day for several reasons; it would prevent the edema which was causing her pain, and by not retaining the fluid this would cut down on nightly trips to the bathroom, noting this process also disrupts the sleep pattern. I also noted her blood pressure was elevated; diuretics are often given to treat high blood pressure. Again, this was another situation where one medication could treat several different issues.

Edema can be a painful process. What happens is when edema is present, the fluid actually causes pressure on the nerves of the lower extremities and this causes pain. When you get rid of the edema and, more importantly, prevent the edema from developing, the pain improves.

This case is a good example on how a chronic painful process can be overlooked, and more importantly, where the fix can be quite simple. Narcotics and NSAIDs are not the only solutions to some painful conditions. Another important fact to understand is NSAIDs often cause or exacerbate edema. They can also cause elevation of the blood pressure. In this case an NSAID would have been the worst thing to give her.

Make sure when you tell your healthcare provider about your problem, that they need to examine, at least that region of the body. I am not sure how edema was missed in this patient over the past few years.

Case Study Number Seven:

A forty-eight year old white female with a several month history of severe headaches, was referred to my office for evaluation and treatment. She was given the diagnosis of "temporal arteritis" (a condition which causes inflammation of the blood vessels of the head). The main clinical presentation of this condition is severe headache. The most serious complication of this condition is acute loss of vision; the ophthalmic artery can become inflamed, and if the blood supply is compromised, blindness can occur. The treatment for this condition is high doses of corticosteroids (prednisone is the most common steroid used to treat this condition). She was taking prednisone for several months; initially 60 mg each morning for a month and her present dose was 40 mg each morning. This is a high dose of steroid, but appropriate for the management of "temporal arteritis," if present. Interestingly enough, in spite of being on such a high dose of prednisone her headaches never really went away. Another interesting fact is that this condition usually causes inflammatory markers in the blood to be elevated, such as, the sedimentation rate and the C-reactive protein, hers were always normal. Patients who have active inflammatory processes which go on for several months (without treatment) tend to get anemic; her blood count was normal. The best way, accurately, to make the diagnosis of temporal arteritis is to do a temporal artery biopsy (a biopsy of the temporal artery done by a surgeon). If the biopsy shows inflammation in the blood vessel, the diagnosis is definitive. However, if the biopsy is negative it is still possible that the condition is present because the inflammation within the blood vessel could skip regions along the blood vessel. It is possible that the biopsy could show a region of non-affected blood vessel and the condition could still be present. She actually did have a biopsy a few months ago and it was negative. Other clinical features which she was experiencing included: a poor sleep pattern, non-restorative sleep process, diffuse muscle tenderness and muscle pain. She was not having any visual disturbances.

Examination revealed an anxious middle-aged white female, who was tender to touch all over. There was no joint swelling. There was right temporal tenderness near the incision from the right temporal artery biopsy site. It should be noted that I asked if she was having right temporal tenderness before the biopsy and she said, "No."

This is where things get interesting. I did not believe she had temporal arteritis; the boat was missed. I explained to her my impression, and that the first order of business was to begin weaning her from the prednisone, as this medication could not be abruptly stopped. The next thing to talk about was what she did have. It was my impression she had fibromyalgia.

I started her on Topamax 25 mg twice a day, with the instruction that the dose should be increased to 50 mg twice a day in one week, if tolerated and not improved. For sleep, I started her on clonazepam 0.5 mg one tablet at bedtime, with the instruction to increase the dose to two tablets at bedtime, if she was not sleeping better after one week.

She returned to the office two weeks later. Her prednisone dose was down to 10 mg each morning. She was feeling much better. She was sleeping better; experienced a restorative sleep pattern and the headaches were almost resolved.

Over the next few weeks the prednisone was tapered to zero and with some minor adjustments of the Topamax, along with some prn (as needed) dosing of Xanax (for anxiety), 0.5 mg tablets (1-3 per day) she was almost symptom free.

Analysis:

This is an important case because it is an excellent example of not only a wrong diagnosis, but also wrong treatment. Unfortunately, patients do not know when doctors miss the boat. This lady was compliant and she did what the doctors told her to do. From a doctor's standpoint, there are many things about the management of this patient, which should have been done differently. First, the diagnosis of temporal arteritis in a forty-eight year old is probably not going to happen. I have been treating people with this condition for over 20 years, and never have seen a person with this condition under the age of sixty; most of these patients are seventy years or older. As a general rule, the inflammatory blood markers are elevated; hers were normal. Second, there was no temporal tenderness and she did get the biopsy. It is possible to get a positive temporal artery biopsy if there is no temporal tenderness, but it is less likely if there is no tenderness at the temporal region. Third, she really did not feel much better on high dose prednisone, even though she was given it for several months. Usually, temporal arteritis responds quickly and nicely (within days) to high doses of prednisone. Unfortunately, the long-term management of this condition with varying doses of steroids is a process, which should be managed by someone experienced with this condition (a rheumatologist), clearly, not the referring physician. Of course, the referring physician was well-intended, but try telling that to the patient. I do not want to sound overly critical. As a rheumatologist, I am expected to understand these conditions and manage them effectively. My only criticism (in this case) with the primary care physician was he should have sought consultation sooner. The patient initially felt better, but not great while on the prednisone. As a general rule, people feel better when taking prednisone, providing they do not experience steroid side effects (weight gain, agitation and fluid retention). There are other potential side effects of steroids, which patients may not be aware of, such as: increased bone turnover leading to low bone mass, increased potential for bruising, increased infection rates, glucose intolerance, cataracts and a potential condition known as avascular necrosis (this can cause bone death; usually at the hip, which may require a hip replacement). This person was exposed to high doses of steroids, for several months, for a condition which did not require steroid treatment.

My initial impression was she had fibromyalgia. The fact she responded to my initial therapy, especially in the face of decreasing doses of steroids, clinched the diagnosis. Most patients with fibromyalgia do not present with headache as the outstanding presentation; the fact was her headache was so intense it led her primary care physician to a diagnosis in which headache is a major manifestation. As the patient, you are at the mercy of your doctor. She was a compliant patient, who went along with the temporal artery biopsy and took high doses of steroids for several months. I am sure many other doctors could have made the same mistake. I do not think the patient could have done anything differently. I have had several other patients, throughout the years, who presented in a similar fashion. However, they were not taking steroids and I was able to sort things out quickly and most importantly, I did not treat them with high doses of steroids for a condition, where it was not necessary.

This is the type of case in which you learn with experience; it is good if the physician develops a steep learning curve with these types of cases.

Case Study Number Eight:

A forty-five year old white female presented with a four year history of achiness, fatigue and occasional irritable bowel. She experienced headaches, easy fatigability, poor memory and poor concentration capacity. She slept well and described a restorative sleep process. Blood work had all been normal, specifically her thyroid function was normal. She stated her primary care doctor encouraged her to try an antidepressant, but she did not want to take an antidepressant; she stated she does not feel depressed. Her past medical history was essentially benign. She only took a few supplements (vitamins) in the morning.

She owned a small medical transcription business, was happily married and had two teenage children (sons) who did well in school and excelled in sports. Between her business and her husband's work they were financially secure.

Examination revealed a well-dressed, middle-aged white female, who appeared younger than her stated age. There was no joint or muscle tenderness. Her examination was normal. She did not appear depressed.

I started this lady on Neurontin 300 mg three times a day. I told her to increase the dose to two tablets three times a day in one week, if there was no improvement. Her follow-up appointment was two weeks later.

When she returned, she told me, she felt the same on the Neurontin 300 mg two tablets three times a day. I told her to increase the dose again, but this time, to take 300 mg three tablets (900mg) three times a day and again increase the dose to 300 mg four tablets (1200 mg) three times a day in a week, if still not improved to a potential daily dose of 3600 mg per day, which is the maximal daily dose of Neurontin (according to the Physician's Desk Reference).

On her follow-up visit, two weeks later she told me that she felt more energetic. Her headaches were improved, less severe, the irritable bowel was less problematic and she was able to remember things and concentrate better. I told her, although I did not feel she was

depressed, she would probably benefit from an antidepressant. I
changed the Neurontin to a 600 mg tablet, two tablets three times a
day (more convenient than the 300 mg tablets). I also started her on
Paxil 10 mg one tablet each morning. I told her to increase the dose to
20 mg each morning in one week, if still not improved.

She returned to the office two weeks later telling me that she was
feeling great, "the best in years." She did increase the Paxil to 20 mg
each morning, another happy camper.

Analysis:

This case is an example of what I would call "atypical fibromyalgia." She had all the classic features of fibromyalgia, but did not have
the sleep pattern abnormalities or the muscle tenderness. This would
be a tough diagnosis to make for most healthcare providers. She did
not fit the classic pattern of fibromyalgia. [Note: Most doctors do not
have an understanding of the typical presentations of fibromyalgia,
let alone the atypical presentations.] Most doctors would have said,
she was depressed or a malingerer. Hypothyroidism was an important
diagnosis to rule out; her thyroid function tests were normal. She did
not appear to be depressed. She certainly had a good marriage, a successful business and her kids were doing well, she seemed to have it all.
What she had, and did not need, was the way she was feeling. It is quite
distressing and demoralizing, to the patient, when they go from doctor
to doctor not feeling well, looking for answers and relief, only to find
that the medical community either thinks they are depressed or crazy.

Unlike the vast majority of patients, with fibromyalgia, a poor sleep
process was not an issue for her. She did not need a sleep aid; a different initial medication approach was needed. There was no inflammation therefore an NSAID would not be appropriate. She was not having
muscle pain therefore a muscle relaxant would not be the answer. This
was the type of patient that should be treated with either one of the
anti-seizure medications (Neurontin, Topamax, or Lyrica) or one of
the SSRI medications (Paxil, Prozac, Zoloft, or Celexa, by no means a

complete list). The combination SSRI/NSRI medications could also be used (Savella, Cymbalta and Effexor). Of these three medications, only the Effexor comes in a generic form. These antidepressants and anti-seizure medications can also be used in combination.

I chose to start with Neurontin. She already had been offered an antidepressant by another doctor, however, for the wrong reason, as she was not depressed. I did not think this class of drug would go over so well on a first visit. I needed to gain some trust first. I also had the feeling she would need combination therapy; therefore, why not start off with the non-antidepressant medication. I chose Neurontin over Lyrica because it was less expensive and many patients do quite well on Neurontin. I did not want to use Topamax (also available as a generic drug) because she was quite thin and weight loss is a common side effect of this medication; a desirable side effect if the patient happens to also be overweight. Note how quickly I advanced the dose of the Neurontin upwards. As a general rule, when I am treating fibromyalgia, I expect patients to respond quickly to the medications. If nothing significant has happened, for the patient, after being on a specific medication at a specific dose after one week, a change has to be made, that is, increase the dose of the medication. If a clinical change has not occurred after one week, it is not going to happen without a medication dose change, or the addition of another medication. I usually will only add the next medication, if the patient is taking the maximum dose of the initial medication and there has been a suboptimal response. Sometimes a medication is helpful, but at higher doses (below the maximum dose) side effects occur. In this situation I may choose to keep the patient at the sub-maximal tolerated dose and add another medication.

After four weeks on the Neurontin, she was up to the maximal dose 600 mg two tablets three times a day. She certainly was much better, but not great. I needed to add another medication to the regimen. By this time, we had developed a good doctor-patient relationship. She recognized I understood her medical condition. She was a pleasant, compliant and reasonable patient. On the third visit, I explained the rationale of adding the antidepressant to her medication regimen; not because of depression, but also for the management of fibromyalgia.

Now she was very receptive to the idea; after all, I was quickly display-
ing a good track record with her, over just three visits. The addition
of Paxil was just what she needed. She continues to do well on this
very effective, inexpensive, totally off-labeled, regimen for the management of her "atypical fibromyalgia."

The take-home message is: fibromyalgia is a constellation of symptoms and clinical findings. Wide spread muscle pain is considered a
major criteria for the diagnosis of this condition. My experience has
shown me, this is not always the case. You could say to me, she just
was really depressed all along and she just was responding to Paxil.
Keep in mind, the first drug I treated her with was the Neurontin, an
anti-seizure medication. This will have no impact on treating primary
depression. The addition of Paxil was the icing on the cake. At the end
of the day, I am not concerned so much with the classification of the
condition, but the management of the condition; call it whatever you
like, I am just out to treat it and make it better.

Case Study Number Nine:

A fifty-four year old Hispanic female referred herself to me for continued management of her fibromyalgia. This condition was diagnosed ten years ago. She was well (ten years ago), until being involved in a motor vehicle accident. She had suffered soft tissue injuries with no broken bones. It was felt that her fibromyalgia was brought on by the motor vehicle accident. It was the other driver's fault. There was litigation and an out-of-court settlement was made. Over the next 3-4 years following the accident, her pain got worse to the degree that she had to go on short-term and then long-term disability. She was treated with a host of NSAIDs, muscle relaxants, antidepressants and anti-seizure medication achieving varying degrees of relief, but she never felt well. She has seen several rheumatologists and pain specialists in the past. She would go from one doctor to the other because she felt that each one was not helping her.

Her clinical features consisted of severe, constant muscle pain and tenderness. She slept poorly and was not refreshed when she awoke in the morning. She had constant headaches, saw several different neurologists and multiple migraine medications were either not helpful or poorly tolerated. Irritable bowel characterized by alternating diarrhea and constipation was problematic and she complained of extreme fatigue.

Her present medication regimen consisted of: Ambien 10 mg at night; Neurontin 600 mg two tablets three times a day; Xanax 2 mg three times a day; Soma 350 mg one tablet three times a day; and most recently Vicodin 5/500 mg one tablet twice a day was added to the medication regimen by her primary care physician. It should be noted, the primary care physician told her, he was only going to give her the one script of Vicodin (60 tablets with no refills).

She told me, Vicodin at one tablet twice a day was not helpful, but when she took two tablets twice a day she would derive 4-5 hours of relief.

Examination revealed a middle-age, Hispanic female who appeared anxious, noting she was quite coherent and responded appropriately to all questions. Global muscle tenderness was present, noting the pain to minimal touch seemed way out of proportion to what I would have expected (an exaggerated response). There was joint tenderness, but no joint swelling. The rest of the examination was normal.

Recent blood work, which included: a complete blood count, comprehensive metabolic profile, thyroid panel and lipid panel were all normal.

Some additional important information is as follows. After three attempts at applying for Social Security disability, with the aid of a disability attorney on her third attempt, she was awarded Social Security disability for her diagnosis of fibromyalgia.

I had her sign a pain contract and performed an in-office urine tox screen, which was consistent with what she was taking. I then advised her to continue with her present medications except, I increased her Vicodin to 10/500 mg with the instructions to take this medication two to three times a day, as needed for pain. I wrote her a script for 90 tablets with no refills and told her to return back to the office in one week.

I saw her one week later, in the office, and she was doing much better. The increased dose of Vicodin was well tolerated. At this visit, I made the decision not to make any other medication changes; I would see her back in three weeks for a follow-up appointment. I will talk more about this case in the analysis. Due to the new FDA acetaminophen guidelines, the Vicodin dose is now 10/325 mg.

Analysis:

This is an important case, which represents a subset of patients with fibromyalgia; patients with this condition, where the use of an opioid is appropriate. This is certainly a judgment call. Opioids should not be the first or second or even third drug used for the management of fibromyalgia, but there are many patients out there, with fibromyalgia, where their only hope for pain relief is with the use of an opioid.

I knew from the first visit, she would require a narcotic for the successful management of her chronic pain. She was a very good historian with regard to all of the previous medications that she used without success. I saw no reason to reinvent the wheel by putting her back on medications which were already failures. She was clearly treated with what I would call conventional therapies. [Note: By conventional therapies, I am talking about medications used which were off-labeled, as I have already discussed earlier.] Also, she did feel better with Vicodin, and I appreciated her honesty in telling me, she was taking more than prescribed from her primary care physician.

In this case, it is clear to see, a narcotic is needed. I did not get the sense she was drug-seeking or doctor shopping. Unfortunately, patients like her are often labeled doctor shoppers. She was just looking for relief. She gave each of the other rheumatologists many months to manage her pain; they were unsuccessful, and she just moved on to someone else with the hope of making progress.

With this case example, I did not get into the specifics regarding each subsequent visit. What I wanted to do here was to point out some basic concepts regarding the management of this type of patient. She was taking a lot of medications, and in spite of it, she still was quite symptomatic. I really did not know what was or was not working. I did know the Vicodin was helpful, when she took two tablets at a time. This would be a good starting point for me. Patients often will feel uncomfortable when they are taking complex medication regimens and major changes are attempted on a first visit. If I increased Vicodin, which I did, and took one or two of the medications away, it is possible that she would have come back a week later feeling worse. I certainly had my eye on trying to cut back or cut out some of her present medications, but not on the first visit. I needed all the other medications to remain at their present doses, while I only adjusted the opioid.

I also chose to see her one week later rather than the usual two week follow-up, from an initial visit. This was because; it does not take long to know where you stand when prescribing any specific dose of an opioid. You will know where you stand with the opioid (at any particular dose) regarding pain relief, after a day or two on the medication. There was no reason to wait two weeks for the response. Also, pain management needs to be done quickly; the medications are either working or they are not, keep in mind the therapeutic response will be dose related.

When she came back a week later, she was doing better, not great, but doing better, we were moving in the right direction. These kinds of cases need careful consideration on what to do next. Keep in mind, she came to me on a complex medication regimen; was still quite symptomatic; and I had to decide which direction to take this. I decided not to make any changes in her medications at the second visit. The reason for this was, I wanted to give her a few weeks of finally feeling better before making any further adjustments, her body needed a rest.

At the next visit (three weeks later), without any further medication changes, from the last visit, she reported to me, she was feeling even better. I attribute this to the fact, her body was able to rest just from the increase in Vicodin; of course, I was sure the other medications were doing their part, too. I just did not know what was doing what. Over the next few months, I was able to reduce some of the doses of the other medications. She continues to do well on her present medication regimen and I see her every two months for a follow-up appointment. Some patients with fibromyalgia need to be managed with narcotics; for these patients it should be the last resort and prior "failed" medication regimens should be well documented in the medical record.

Case Study Number Ten:

A forty-three year old white female presents to my office for evaluation of fatigue, muscle pain, joint pain (without swelling) and episodes of headache. She does not sleep well and is not rested when she wakes up. She has seen multiple doctors (neurologist, rheumatologist, psychiatrist and internists). She stated that nobody is listening to her and she feels abandoned by the medical community.

Her past medical history is significant for high blood pressure, which is well controlled on Dyazide (a diuretic) 37.5/25 mg one tablet per day, hypothyroidism for which she takes Levothyroxine 0.88 micrograms a day (her thyroid function is normal on this dose of medication) and anxiety for which she takes Xanax 1mg two to three times a day, on an as needed basis.

She has three teenage sons and is divorced. She has been married three times. She works at home doing some type of Internet business.

When I asked about her visit to the psychiatrist, she told me, she only saw her once, and was told there was no need to return, "I'm normal."

Examination revealed an overweight middle-aged female, who was nicely dressed. She seemed a bit anxious. Her examination was significant for diffuse muscle tenderness, no joint swelling nor joint range of motion deficit; otherwise, no abnormalities were identified. Basic blood work was normal.

After the examination, I asked her what she thought the problem was, after all, the other doctors she saw had no clue, perhaps she had the answer. Her response was, "You tell me, you're the doctor." I told her, it is possible that she may have a condition called fibromyalgia. She told me, "Fibromyalgia is a condition that doctors give people when they don't know what's wrong with you." I asked her, if she ever has read about fibromyalgia and she said, "Yes." I then asked her if she thought, based on her readings, her symptoms, and for the lack of any other diagnosis at this time, if she thought it was possible she had this condition. She did not say much in response to my question.

I asked if she ever had depression and she quickly responded, "No." Over the past two years, she has had three different primary care physicians. She was taking no other medications than what she already listed.

I told her, I thought she may have fibromyalgia. I was willing to try to help her, but she would have to be on board with the diagnosis, otherwise, I did not think I would be able to help her. I cannot effectively manage a patient, if they think they have a different condition than what I am attempting to treat. I told her, she could consider a third rheumatology opinion, as I was the second. When I asked her what the first rheumatologist thought she had, her response was, "I didn't like him; he was rude."

I told her, I wanted to start her on a sleep aid and to see how she responds to this type of medication. She then went on to tell me that she had tried several sleep aids in the past, which were not successful (Ambien, Lunesta, trazadone and amitriptyline).

I told her, I would like to try nortriptyline (a tricyclic antidepressant) which often is quite helpful for sleep. She agreed to do this. I started her on 25 mg at night and advised her to increase the dosage to two tablets at night (50 mg) in one week, if not improved. Her follow-up appointment was in two weeks.

When she returned, she told me, there was some improvement in her sleep and muscle pain on the nortriptyline at 25 mg at bedtime, but she was drowsy in the morning, when she took 50 mg of the medication. She went back to the 25 mg dose at night. I told her, we should try adding Neurontin to the regimen, 300 mg three times a day (the last dose at night). I told her to return in two weeks.

At the time of her next visit, she stated, she was feeling a bit better, but was very concerned about taking, "Too much medication;" she cut the Neurontin back to one tablet twice a day instead of three times a day. She spent most of the visit telling me, all I wanted to do was to give her more medication, and I was not addressing the basis of her problem. She then asked me about "holistic" (natural) remedies which, she learned about through the Internet. After about a half-hour of going around in circles, she told me, she did not want to take any medication. I told her that would be fine, if that was her preference. I would see her on an as-needed basis. I also suggested, and documented in the medical record, she should get another opinion from another rheumatologist. I never saw her again, oh well.

Analysis:

I had to include this Case Study in the book. Believe it or not, I seem to get a lot of people like this: the ones who feel abandoned by the medical community, nobody understands them, and ironically, after bending over backwards for them, they really do not want anything. What is going on here? I really do think it goes beyond their concern about taking medication; after all, what else were they expecting? The history is very important. This patient was certainly making the rounds with the medical community. These types of patients always seem to see multiple doctors, but never come to the office with medical records. It would be interesting to know what the psychiatrist thought. It was interesting; she had been on many of the medications which are used to treat fibromyalgia. She was vague on who in the past had prescribed them to her.

I try to be as objective, as possible, with every new patient. I want to give people the benefit of the doubt. I am pretty good at figuring people out on a first visit. When a patient has gone to multiple specialists; has been treated with various medications without improvement; and feels nobody understands them; I like to believe that perhaps everyone else did get it wrong. Perhaps the medical community has let this patient fall through the cracks. I am willing to work with them and embrace their story.

Things did not seem to add up here from the start, but I was willing to go down the path with her, but only so far. As you can see; we did not get too far. In the end, she was actually resistant to the concept of treatment. It is absurd because she came to me for help. What did she really want? I do not know if these patients have psychiatric problems or perhaps it is about attention, I am not sure. Perhaps it is just sport for these people. I suspect, this person will be making appointments, to see other people, and the cycle will continue. Some people like to be the victim.

Sometimes it is not about the doctors getting it wrong; it is the patient. I get quite candid with these people. When they say to me, "I'm sorry for wasting your time;" I reply to them by saying, "It's not a waste of my time;" I am trying to help them. They need to understand, this is what I do. I have an obligation to be in their face, if need be. I like to think that the buck stops at my office. I do not want to waste the patient's time or money. There seems to be an endless number of patients, who want to be seen by me and other rheumatologists. Sometimes these patients are happy to have a diagnosis, and for whatever the reason, they just do not want to take a medication. I tell these patients, nobody dies from fibromyalgia. They probably just will continue to be miserable and live an uncomfortable life, if not treated. I always leave the door open for these patients, however, they usually never return.

Case Study Number Eleven:

A seventy year old white female, retired seamstress, presents with a six year history of progressive pain, numbness and hypersensitivity over the region of the right upper lateral thigh. Her symptoms were gradual in onset, but have been more problematic over the past eighteen months. At times, the pain and burning sensation, over this region, is quite debilitating and other times, it is a dull and nagging sensation; but it is always present. In earlier years, the symptoms were intermittent. At times just the sensation of her five year old grandson's hand brushing up against her right upper lateral thigh was enough to send her through the roof.

Her past medical history is significant for hypothyroidism, non-insulin dependent diabetes, hypertension (high blood pressure) and she had a complete hysterectomy at the age of fifty-one. The above mentioned conditions are all well controlled on medication.

Examination was significant for a normal blood pressure, obesity (her weight was 197 pounds), non-tender osteoarthritic hand and foot changes were evident and there was a small amount of edema at her ankles. The right upper lateral thigh displayed decreased sensitivity to pin prick compared to the left side and light touch over this region was exquisitely tender; noting that firm pressure applied to the upper lateral, right thigh did not elicit discomfort. The rest of the examination was otherwise unremarkable.

I started the patient on Neurontin 300 mg one tablet three times a day and told her if the medication was well tolerated, and she was not improved in one week, she should increase the medication to 300 mg two tablets three times a day. The follow-up appointment would be in two weeks.

Two weeks later, she returned stating that she was doing much better; she was taking two tablets three times a day. There was much less discomfort, over the right upper lateral thigh region; the heightened sensitivity to light touch was gone (no further lightning bolts when her grandchild touched her thigh); the medication was well tolerated and she was quite pleased with the results. I will see her in four months for a follow-up appointment or sooner, if needed.

Analysis:

This is an example of a very common problem that many people experience. This is a painful neuropathy called Meralgia Paresthetica. This is an impingement neuropathy (the nerve is being pressed), and the problem usually is coming from nerve irritation at the level of the lumbar region (specifically the nerve roots of the second and third lumbar vertebrae as they exit the spinal region and this explains this process 90 percent of the time). Ten percent of the time, the nerve irritation has a peripheral origin. This means the point of nerve irritation occurs at a distance away from the lower spinal region. The most common peripheral location for this nerve irritation occurs at the inner, lower waist region. This is where the nerve surfaces, to provide sensation to the upper lateral thigh region. The nerve roots of L2 and L3 combine to form the lateral femoral cutaneous nerve. Irritation of this nerve causes the lateral femoral cutaneous nerve syndrome, also known as Meralgia Paresthetica. Sometimes, this can be the first presentation of hypothyroidism, so in the work-up, thyroid function needs to be evaluated. Even if a patient has known and treated hypothyroidism, the thyroid function has to be evaluated to make sure that the patient is getting adequate replacement.

Painful neuropathies can significantly affect a person's day-to-day activities; they are painful. The peripheral etiology (10% of the time) can be related to obesity; the excess body fat hangs over the region where the nerve comes to the surface causing pressure on the nerve and hence creating the symptoms. Sometimes weight reduction can be the solution. Also, wearing tight clothing around the waist can cause pressure on the nerve, and this, too, can cause the symptoms to occur. In certain cases of peripheral origin, a steroid injection to the upper medial thigh region may be helpful. The lumbar origin process may also be responsive to an injection, but both of these procedures need to be done by an experienced specialist, usually an anesthesiologist or physiatrist who specializes in pain management. In this situation (regarding this patient) a medication approach was employed.

Sometimes an NSAID may be helpful, especially if at the point of nerve irritation, there is inflammation, such as, the lower back, where there may be an associated degenerative arthritic change which is irritating the nerve. Most often, NSAIDs do not work well for the management of this condition. Since this is a neuropathy, it needs to be treated with medication which is used to treat neuropathic pain. Medications which are helpful for the management of neuropathic pain include Neurontin, Topamax, Lyrica, and Lamictal. This is an off-labeled use of these medications with regard to the management of Meralgia Paresthetica. I have used all of these medications, for the management of this condition, and each one has been effective (different patients respond to these medications differently). The response, to the medication, will also be dose dependent; some patients respond to a lower dose while others need to be on higher doses.

The bottom line is: this is a very common condition, which I see in my office. Usually, this problem is not even the main problem for which they are seeing me. The good news is, the condition does have a name and a treatment and most patients respond well to one of the three medications named above. Many patients tell me, previous healthcare providers have told them, nothing can be done for a painful neuropathy. This is not exactly true. Perhaps there may be no "cure" for the neuropathic process, but there is certainly treatment which can address the pain without the use of NSAIDs or a narcotic. This is true!

five

Pre-Authorization

If you think healthcare coverage means all your healthcare needs are being covered, you are clearly mistaken. I hope I am not the one who has to break this news to you (for those of you who are fortunate enough to have health insurance). Many have health insurance, but have such high co-pays and deductibles; it is almost like not having insurance at all! In many cases, there are certain medications, your doctor may want you to take, which your insurance company will not cover. In order for you to get that medication there is a procedure of paperwork and sometimes telephone conversations that your doctor and his/her staff has to go through to get it approved by the insurance company. This process is called pre-authorization. The same process oftentimes has to be obtained for certain diagnostic procedures, such as, MRI's, CT scans, nuclear medicine studies, and referrals to see specialists.

When a pre-authorization request is made from the healthcare provider's office, there are insurance company guidelines regarding when a drug is approved or disapproved. If a request for a specific medication is made, the insurance company is going to want supporting documentation as to the medical necessity for the request. After doing this for so many years, I know when it is appropriate to make such a request. Remember, what I am about to say (as this will help you down the line), should you find yourself in the situation where a pre-authorization for a medication, any medication, is required.

The medication that is being requested has to be FDA approved for the condition being treated. If the medication is being used in an off-labeled fashion, then forget about it because it will be denied. I think there may be a two-fold explanation for denial when trying to get pre-authorization for a medication being used in an off-labeled fashion. When a request for a pre-authorization of a medication is made, you know the medication is not cheap; I am sure there is a financial component to the equation. Also, if a patient were to have a severe adverse reaction to the medication, which is being used in an off-labeled manner, I assume there may be a liability issue for the insurance company, for being involved with the procurement of the medication. When medical malpractice cases occur, all parties involved are sued and the plaintiff's (the person who is suing) attorney is looking for all the deep pockets to pay up. I think it is fair to say, insurance companies have bigger pockets than the liability coverage the healthcare provider carries.

After medical appropriateness of the medication is determined, the insurance plan wants to know what other similar medications were tried (or avoided) and the reason for their avoidance or failure. If the initial medication, which was prescribed was generic, and the new drug being requested is not generic; and other similar class generic medications are available, the insurance plan will deny the request, specifically stating one of the other generic medications needs to be tried first. Insurance companies may have different specific rules on their protocols for getting approval for pre-authorization of a medication. For example, an insurance plan may carry a specific class of medication, such as NSAIDs, which may have seven different generics within that medication class. Some insurance plans will state the patient needs to fail two or three other medications, in that class, before the pre-authorization will be approved. Other insurance plans may state "all" the generic medications in that class have to be tried and failed before the pre-authorization will be approved.

Now, there may be a situation where a medication needs to be pre-approved from the get-go because other medications, in that particular class, would be contraindicated to prescribe; the following is an example. Let us say an elderly man, comes to see me, who has an arthritic right knee, painful with some swelling. He needs an NSAID. However, he has a cardiac condition known as atrial fibrillation. Because of this abnormal heart rhythm he needs to be on the blood thinner warfarin (Coumadin). This medication thins the blood and can be associated with an increased risk of bleeding. Well, as you now already know, NSAIDs can be associated with increased bleeding risk. I still want to give this person an NSAID, not just because of the knee arthritis, but because of other areas of symptomatic arthritis, including his hands and neck. The NSAID which would be the safest to prescribe to this elderly man on warfarin is Celebrex. Remember, Celebrex does not increase bleeding time and is less likely to irritate the gastric mucosa, at least in theory. [Note: From my observation with patients in this situation, I would say this is true.] Keep in mind, I am not just concerned about bleeding when prescribing an NSAID; as already mentioned, there are other potential adverse effects which have to be considered when prescribing NSAIDs to patients of all ages, and especially when other complex medical conditions coexist.

With regard to getting a pre-authorization for a medication, this is a relatively simple task for the doctor to accomplish, in most circumstances. If the healthcare provider fills out the necessary paperwork, which should take less than a minute, the office staff can fill in the rest of the information, such as, patient identification number, address, and date of birth. If the doctor, using our seventy-two year old patient, as an example, just takes a minute to write down, "seventy-two year old male with a-fib (atrial fibrillation) on warfarin needing Celebrex for knee pain and swelling, all other NSAIDs contraindicated;" this should be a slam dunk for the patient. The request should not be denied. If it is, I will get on the phone and call the medical director, usually a sixty second conversation in favor of the patient, or I might just have to dictate a letter to the appeals committee, a process which takes me 60 seconds to do, too.

Very rarely, the insurance company will play hardball and tell me they want to have a phone conference with me, with their committee on the other end. Now, in this situation, this is quite disruptive to my practice. They usually schedule this phone conference at 9:00 AM, it may certainly be convenient for them but not for me. By this time of day, I am already seeing patients and probably running late. This phone conversation is certainly not going to help me with time management. They also tell you during the notification process that I do not have to participate in the conference. By the way, with these phone conferences, the patient is also given the opportunity to participate. I do believe this is a technique of wearing down the physician. I can assure you, the patient would not have a prayer in the world of winning the argument without my participation. The fact of the matter is, I am the expert in the field of rheumatology, I know what is appropriate for my patients and I know how to play the insurance company game. They are the ones who make the guidelines. Whenever I request a pre-authorization, I am doing so in the context of what the insurance company mandates. What I find interesting and quite frankly "amusing" is when I am making an appeal, by phone to a review committee, not even one of the committee members is a rheumatologist! I am supposed to be asking permission to do something for a patient from people who are not a specialist in my field!

These committees are composed of various people, non-medical personal, pharmacists, and usually a doctor, who no longer sees patients and is practicing administrative medicine. Do not get me wrong, I am not criticizing these doctors, they play an important role in the organization of the healthcare plan. I do think this protocol practice is, in part, designed to take the healthcare provider to the limit and try, in part, to wear them out. I recently had a patient who needed a very expensive medication to treat an arthritic condition which was not responding to a step-wise fashion of treatment. I needed to take therapy to the next level. I really do not think any board certified rheumatologist would have disagreed with my next plan of action. The medication was denied, I sent a letter of appeal, and a 9:00 AM conference was scheduled.

This phone meeting took 30 minutes; I had the patient explain her story to the committee, the medical problem and treatment failures, and then I took the reins and pleaded "our" case. At the end, when I was talking to the doctor, I made the comment, "Since you're a rheumatologist what would you do?" I knew this doctor was not a rheumatologist; otherwise, this meeting would not even have taken place! By this time, 25 minutes into the meeting, (keeping in mind that when the call came into my office I was already busy in my exam room seeing a patient); I even kept the door open so this patient could hear me doing battle with the insurance company (a modern day David versus Goliath). Patient confidentiality was maintained.

I wanted the patient in the exam room to get a taste of what doctors have to do for their patients behind the scenes. Also, my waiting room is filling up, and quite frankly, I was quite ticked off that this conversation even lasted this long; I thought it would go 10 minutes max. At this point in time, I had only one option, to turn this into sport; I am going hunting! The doctor on the other end of the phone then told me that she was an endocrinologist; I almost fell off my chair. Not to be condescending, I was not worried about the other members of the committee, I knew much more about the condition at hand and the appropriate treatments. It was now time for me to shame the endocrinologist, in a nice and respectful way; the last thing I wanted to do was to undermine the plight of the patient. Needless to say, this was a short conversation. My final thoughts to the committee were, if they had a better suggestion, with an alternative more cost effective plan, I would certainly embrace their recommendation. That very afternoon, I received notification that the medication was approved. I was going to be the best advocate for my patient I possibly could, regardless of the obstacles placed in my path. As a physician, it is important to fight these battles not just because it is in the best interest of the patient; but I do believe that if an insurance company gets to know you as a straight shooter and one who plays by the book that "they wrote," they are less likely to be a wall the next time you come knocking.

Although this process was frustrating and time consuming and irritated me for the rest of the day, not to mention all of the explaining to the rest of the patients whose appointments were delayed by the phone conference, it was a good investment of time and I did get my patient what was needed. I also get to tell this story to the reader giving them insight into the pre-authorization process, which I think is important to understand, especially if you find yourself in this situation; a real possibility.

It is extremely rare for a medication to ultimately be denied after having gone through the protocol, which I have already outlined. Sometimes I get to the end of the road, with how far I can take the patient, with the pre-authorization process. The patient then has the option of taking this process further, such as legal action in which I have never had a patient go that far, or they may have to settle for a medication which is inferior to what I initially had intended. I guess "second rate therapy" is better than "no therapy" at all.

My only suggestion to the patient is, if you find yourself in a situation whereby your doctor's office informs you, they are in the process of going through the motions of attempting to get a pre-authorization of a medication, procedure, or consultant referral, be patient because this can be quite a frustrating process for the doctor's office. At least you have a doctor that is trying to be an advocate in your best interest!

six

Doctor-Patient Relationship

The doctor-patient relationship is an important relationship, especially when a chronic condition is being managed. If you have a condition where you need to see your doctor on a regular basis, you had better like and get along with your doctor. I have had patients, who I have been following on a regular basis for over two decades. I have known their children, when they were in diapers and now these children are grown, married, and have children of their own. I have been in longer relationships with my patients than many have had with their own marriages. In some ways, the doctor-patient relationship is like a marriage. Throughout the years, I have gotten to know many intimate details about my patient's personal and family lives; about workplaces and family dynamics. Certainly, I am not trying to be intrusive, but a lot of stress and anxiety, which has a key role in chronic pain issues, is based around the family nucleus and to effectively treat the patient as a whole these issues need to come to light and be addressed. There has to be a level of trust and confidence that the patient feels with the doctor.

In my medical practice, there is a spectrum of patients whom I follow. I have a following of patients that have been under my care for

229

a few decades, others for ten or more years, another group of people for five or more years, less than five years, and of course I regularly see new patients. New relationships are developed on a daily basis. This is an important chapter which I want to put out there for the reader. I believe it will be quite helpful for you.

This chapter goes towards the concept of being a good patient and trying to develop a good relationship with your healthcare provider. I intend to be honest with my readers, and I want them to know, what and how doctors think. If the patient becomes too much of a burden to the doctor, by what is perceived to be disruptive to the practice, the patient runs the risk of being discharged from the care of that physician. This will certainly create a new set of problems for the patient. Some doctors want to see medical records from previous healthcare providers before accepting a new patient. If the medical record documents the patient was a problem, they may not accept that person into their practice.

Aside from whatever issues there may be that are inherent with the patient (whether perceived by others or not), there are other major hurdles which have to be jumped with regard to finding a healthcare provider who can appropriately manage fibromyalgia or other chronic painful conditions.

Depending on where a person lives will dictate what is available to them regarding treatment. If a person lives in a small town, it is unlikely there will be a chronic pain specialist. Big cities usually have pain specialists. Even if you eventually get to the right person, who has the skill to deliver the appropriate treatment, there is the factor of the patient and provider meshing well together. I can tell within five minutes whether I will be able to get along with a new patient. On a weekly basis, I evaluate a new patient, who presents with anger and hostility towards me; they usually have not even given me enough time to piss them off! I sometimes have to cut the visit short and tell the patient, I do not think we are going to work well together, and they need to find another doctor. Sometimes, I will point blank tell the person within a few minutes, into the visit, they seem angry and hostile, and I understand their frustration, and I want our relationship to work out. This usually changes the tone of the visit (for the better), and we are able to productively move forward.

It is important to start off on the right foot with the person, who will be providing pain management (or with any doctor for that matter). Remember, you are the one with the problem. Most doctors, who manage chronic pain, are quite busy with lots of patients, and they have a steady supply of new patients just waiting to be seen. My attitude, and I am sure one shared by many other providers, is, I am too busy to have to deal with attitude and confrontation with a new patient. I want to help people, but I am not going to be uncomfortable with a patient in my own office. I do not need to put up with any abuse. I am respectful to my patients and they need to be reasonable with me; it works both ways. I say this to you because if you are that patient, who has been through the mill, with other doctors in the past, and feel you have been abandoned by the medical community, you need to drop those feelings off at the door and be friendly and positive, if you really want the pain management specialist to embrace your pain issues.

Do not raise any red flags on the first visit. It is much easier for a doctor to say at the end of the first visit, they cannot help you and you need to go somewhere else. A true doctor-patient relationship, during the first visit, has not been established yet. The doctor has no obligation to render treatment. It is more difficult to drop an established patient, especially if they are on a complex pain medication regimen. The doctor cannot just abandon the patient, but a hostile or non-compliant patient can be discharged from the practice, with instructions to see another pain specialist, or return back to their primary care physician to seek further instructions. The pain specialist will need to give a certain amount of medication refills, but after that the patient will have to take it upon themselves to find another doctor to assume their care.

In general, doctors do not like to drop patients, but they will do it if they must. When I have an established patient and I feel that tension is developing, I like to have a candid discussion about what is going on. I want to know where the problem lies; did I do or say something that irritated the patient? Is there displaced anger? There are lots of reasons why a patient could be angry. I find the best way to figure this out, is to just ask the question point blank, I will get a direct answer. Let us just cut to the chase and move forward. The majority of the time these issues can be quickly resolved and we move forward; sometimes we have to part ways. I will always try to work things out with established patients. Since we are on the subject of disgruntled patients, I do have to tell you a true story, you be the judge.

About 14 years ago, a well off, elderly woman who was seventy-eight years old came to my office for evaluation and treatment of degenerative arthritis of the hands. This really was quite a straightforward case. I do need to give you a description of this lady. She was nicely dressed, clearly well educated, well spoken, and she was accompanied by her distinguished looking elderly husband. They were from the upper west side of New York City. They also had a home in Tucson. The management of her arthritic hands was simple. I had sent her for baseline blood work and noticed that she had a mild anemia (low blood count). On her follow-up visit (two weeks later) I explained to her the findings on her blood work, and further studies needed to be done to determine the cause of the anemia. Keep in mind, aside from her arthritic hands she felt quite well, and had no other medical complaints.

I sent her for iron studies and Hemoccult studies (the Hemoccult studies are a series of three cards which test the stool for blood). It turned out that all three Hemoccult cards were positive for the presence of blood. What this meant was she was losing blood from somewhere in the gastrointestinal tract. The source of bleeding needed to be determined. I sent her to see a gastroenterologist. He performed a colonoscopy on her and identified a tumor in a portion of her large bowel which turned out to be malignant (colon cancer). She was then referred to a surgeon, who was able to completely cut out the cancer and she was cured. She had no surgical or post-surgical complications, and did not require chemotherapy or radiation therapy. She did not require a permanent or temporary colostomy. It really was a good catch on my part; by finding the cancer early her life was saved. Had I taken the attitude that she was probably anemic because she was just an elderly patient, she would have certainly died from colon cancer.

This patient had a follow-up appointment with me six weeks after her colon surgery. I was running late that day (like most days), and when I finally got to see her I was 40 minutes late for her appointment. There is a reason I have cable television in the waiting room; it does make the time pass more quickly. If I am running late, at least by the time I get to the patient, they will be up to snuff on the news of the day. I always apologize to my patients when I am running late. They all know I do not like to rush people and I take care of what needs to be addressed, and then some. It is not difficult to run behind in the office. Here is what happened with this lady. She was very angry with me that I ran late. I tried to make the most of the visit. I thought she would be delighted to see me; after all, I was responsible for saving her life. I could not believe her attitude and what I was hearing. A week later, I received a nasty letter from her about her having to wait 40 minutes for her follow-up appointment, and she was not coming back to see me anymore! You decide; so much for gratitude! I have plenty of stories that I can tell, but this one takes the cake!

It is important to understand that doctors do not like to run late. Some are very good at keeping on schedule; these are the ones who see patients every 10-15 minutes and have no time to talk about more than one or two issues. I cannot practice that way. What patients do not realize is that as the day progresses (and I am running behind later and later) I want to get out of the office too, as quickly as possible. I need an hour break at lunchtime, not necessarily to eat lunch, but to clear my desk for the second part of the day. I use that time to call back patients; refill prescriptions; go through my mail; go to the bank (a medical practice is a business); there are plenty of things that need to be done throughout the day. What does not get done during the lunch hour needs to be done at the end of the day and this will be in addition to whatever accumulates during the afternoon. Just understand, there is more to what goes on in the doctor's office than what appears on the surface. Be patient, be nice, and you will get what you need. Remember, in today's medical climate there are a lot of procedures, tests, and medications which need special approval from the insurance company (a process I discussed in great detail in a specific section of this book titled Pre-Authorization). Doctors do not like having to jump through hoops for ungrateful and difficult patients. Position yourself, in a relationship with a doctor, where they want to bend over backwards for you and take your needs to the mat. I always get great satisfaction when I have a nice patient who needs me to do battle with an insurance company, and I am able to get approved what is needed for the patient. This is a real relationship builder. Strong relationships between the doctor and patient are important for the management of challenging medical conditions.

While we are on the subject of keeping the relationship between you and your doctor strong, let me give you some helpful tidbits of advice. Try not to call your doctor on a weekend for the refill of a maintenance medication. Of course, there are always reasons why people may need to have a script refilled over the weekend. If a call comes to me, on a weekend, involving the request for a non-narcotic medication refill, I will call back the patient and patiently listen to the circumstance for the weekend request. If it is an appropriate weekend request, I will call it into the pharmacy and not make an issue about it with the patient. I realize that medical problems do not just occur Monday through Friday, 8:00 AM -5:00PM (my office hours). I do not mind a weekend phone call, if it is legitimate. I have had patients call me on a weekend, just to ask me non-urgent questions just because it was a convenient time for them to contact me (this really is true); I think you will agree, this is not an appropriate weekend call.

The only reason why I mention weekend and/or after hour requests to you, is because doctors prefer to conduct medical business during an office visit and during office hours. We want to have a medical chart in front of us every time we communicate with a patient. Whenever I get a call outside of office hours, I have to document that communication on a separate piece of paper, and then I have to place it in the medical record when I get back to the office. Patients do not realize what goes on behind the scenes of their phone calls. Do not make it a habit to keep calling doctors out of hours. It will contribute to lowering the "discharge from the practice threshold" if the relationship should begin to tarnish with time. Remember, with chronic pain management, aside from getting the medication regimen right, it is all about the doctor-patient relationship. Do your part to keep it healthy.

Opioid management guidelines, in any given practice, will usually be outlined in the pain contract. If you are not sure how a doctor likes to do certain things just ask, "What is your policy about . . . ?" Things will go well between the patient and the doctor when there is mutual respect and understanding. Some doctors may have specific ways or quirks about the way they do things; try to figure this out. I am not telling you to be subservient, just position yourself in a way in which your best interests will be served.

While on the subject of the doctor-patient relationship, something should also be mentioned about doctor-doctor relationships. Primary care physicians have their own preference to which specialist they refer their patients. Not all doctors like each other, I am sure this goes for all lines of work. I always ask a patient, when they initially come to see me, who their primary care doctor is and how they found out about me. When they tell me the name of a doctor, who usually does not refer to me, that tells me they were initially sent somewhere else, and the patient had to search me out on their own. Sometimes patients feel uncomfortable about even disclosing this information (of being sent somewhere else and then eventually finding their way to me on their own). With all honesty, sometimes a patient comes to see me for an initial visit, and for whatever the reason we do not click, and we never see each other again; this is best for both of us in the long run. It is very important to establish a healthy bond between the patient and the physician on the first visit. First impressions are important, go with them.

By the time most patients get to see me, they are at their wits end. They have been through the mill and around the block, a process which in many instances has been going on for years. I want the relationship to work. I want to make that connection and I will outright validate their journey and tell them I want to help them, and will be diligent in my approach to their pain management. Encouragement and reassurance can go a long way. I have to treat the mind and body as a whole. It is an interesting phenomenon when I sit down with a patient for the first time; listen to them (and I mean really listen to them); examine them; validate the problem; outline a plan of action and then they tell me nobody else has ever taken the time to be so thorough with them. They specifically tell me they now have a sense that somebody cares about their condition and is willing to work with them. I do believe, the patient has to feel you are in control, know what you are doing, and have a track record of success. They need this to move forward with a positive attitude.

How is it patients can walk into my office for an initial visit, many expressing anger, certainly misdirected at me, as I just met them, shed some tears, and at the end of the visit tell me they are already beginning to feel better? I have not physically done anything yet, I have only outlined a strategy for the management of their condition. It all boils down to hope; many of these patients have lost hope. They feel disenfranchised and abandoned by the medical community; many, who come to see me, initially feel this is going to be just another visit and an exercise in futility. It is my job to breathe new life into an old dead problem.

I do believe appropriate management of fibromyalgia goes beyond the prescribing of medications. The practitioner also has to be a coach, advocate, supporter, and in some circumstances play the role of a therapist. I often have to get into personal issues, not to be intrusive, but to get to the root of certain factors in their home or work life that could be significantly affecting their chronic pain and fibromyalgia symptomatology. I often have a patient, who comes in for a follow-up appointment, complaining of increased pain stating that the medications are no longer working or that they want me to increase their pain medication. By spending a bit more time talking about their family and social issues, I can usually identify a problem which needs to be addressed in a non-pharmacological way. I particularly go down this path when a patient, comes for a follow-up appointment with new pain issues, who at the time of their last visit, was doing quite well on their medication regimen.

Clearly, aside from the actual medication regimen, which will be necessary to deliver the patient from their chronic pain, you will also need your doctor, just like the climbers of Mt. Everest need their Sherpa guides to reach their destination. In both situations, a very important relationship of mutual trust and understanding has to be established for the team to safely and successfully reach their ultimate goal.

seven

What Have We Learned?

There has been a lot of information presented in this book. By now, the reader should have a much better understanding of fibromyalgia and other chronic painful conditions, but most importantly, know there is effective and affordable treatment for these conditions. It is unacceptable for anyone to have to suffer with chronic pain; this does not have to be the case.

I have talked about a host of medications, which may be quite helpful as a drug therapy when prescribed as either a single agent or in combination. The reader, by now, should understand that fibromyalgia is a real medical condition, which can be quite debilitating, if not well managed. The concept of off-labeling medications for the management of chronic painful conditions and fibromyalgia is a key concept towards achieving maximal pain control.

Unfortunately, the patient cannot go it alone, when trying to obtain relief from these painful conditions, as the participation of the healthcare provider is essential. The reader now should know exactly who they need to see; you know what to look for in a healthcare provider, who supposedly embraces chronic pain patients. You now have the ability to quickly determine if the healthcare provider is going to be the right fit for you. You should also have the understanding where not to go; and should you find yourself at the wrong medical office, how to extricate yourself from there as quickly and efficiently as possible. You now have a sound understanding of how to interact with healthcare providers; how to make the most of an office visit; and what is necessary to build a good doctor-patient relationship. The concept of the pain contract and urine drug testing is important for both the patient and physician; you will need to adhere, graciously, to this policy.

In my opinion, there are plenty of available, inexpensive generic medications for the management of fibromyalgia and other chronic painful conditions. You just need to associate yourself with a doctor, who takes on these types of patients; they are out there. The vast majority of patients can be helped. They can live normal and productive lives. They can maintain jobs; enjoy their families and free time; and most importantly can carry on living a meaningful existence.

Finally, I really do have to give thanks to my patients as they stuck with me, throughout the years, as my learning curve was growing. I have learned a great deal from them, as well as, from other doctors along the way. The attending physicians, through my rise from internship, residency, and finally fellowship have all contributed to my growth and development as a doctor. I still can remember valuable teachings, from over 20 years ago, which seems like it was just yesterday. Doctors learn their craft in many ways: textbooks, journals, lectures, residency training programs, and from other doctors on a one-on-one basis. The take-home message for the reader is, there is a lot to know in the field of medicine and nobody knows it all. It is up to each individual doctor to continue to educate themselves after formal medical training has been completed. We can learn a lot from our patients, as I have, with regard to managing fibromyalgia and other chronic painful conditions.

Medicine is far from being an exact science; that is why we call it the "practice" of medicine. The word practice may be unsettling to some, who wants to be practiced on? Remember, practice makes perfect, and "experts," in any area of life in general, practice all the time. Practice should not be such a scary word to the patient.

I believe if you have read this book (and I have written it in a way that should be understood by everyone), you should be in a much better position to go out there and begin your journey towards getting the proper treatment you require. Just remember, the key points in this book and it should take you far. Share the information you have learned with your healthcare provider, and begin to take the journey together. Your success will depend on your determination and the constructive partnership you forge with your treating physician. I wish all of you well.

Epilogue

Today, for those healthcare providers, who even believe in the diagnosis of fibromyalgia, it is felt to be a rheumatologist's condition to manage. It is a sad state of affairs to know that many rheumatologists will not even see a fibromyalgia patient. I also find it interesting to note, I would say the most common diagnosis in my practice is fibromyalgia and chronic pain. Between these two conditions, this makes up about 60%-70% of my medical practice. Keeping in mind, fibromyalgia is felt to belong to the rheumatologist; I found it astounding, when I took my initial rheumatology Board Certification Exam in the 1990's, and even a few years ago, when I took my Recertification Exam, I can remember only one question on fibromyalgia. Of course, for a very rare condition called Multicentric Reticulohistiocytosis, which I have only seen in textbooks, there were five questions about this condition on the Board Exam, go figure! Even the people, who are supposed to be the experts on fibromyalgia (rheumatologists), are minimally tested by the Board of Internal Medicine on the topic of fibromyalgia. I do have a theory for this, and I believe because the management of fibromyalgia is so subjective, and really it is such a grey zone of medicine, the Board of Internal Medicine is not going to ask any question(s) on fibromyalgia, which would be considered more complex than the most basic concept. Any question on the Board Exam regarding the topic of fibromyalgia, which ventures into subjectivity would cause uproar from the doctors taking the test, especially if they failed the test by one question, which often happens!

The purpose of this book is to validate chronic pain and fibromyalgia, and to assist the patient in moving towards the right direction for appropriate treatment. I want to be able to streamline the process for effective and appropriate pain management. I am hopeful that I will save the patient time, money, added frustration, and send them in the right direction for effective management. There is plenty of affordable medication which is available for chronic pain management. You just have to move in the right direction, the right path begins with the pages in this book.

I realize I cannot single handedly manage everyone out there with chronic pain; certainly this is not my intention. However, it is my goal to connect with the general public, to the masses of people out there, who are suffering from chronic painful conditions. I do realize there is a dilemma to writing this book. This book is geared to the general public, however, the concepts and principles of this book need to mediated and facilitated by the healthcare provider. I have taken great care to explain things in a way which the general public and healthcare provider will understand. I have written this book in the same language I use when I speak to my patients. Everything I have said in this book is exactly what I have said to my patients throughout the years. I thought it would be great, if I could take all of my experience with the management of chronic painful conditions and put it into a source (a book) where people could read about it and connect with what I have to say. It turns out there are a lot of people, out there, who not only suffer from chronic pain, but also many suffer from the same types of painful conditions (of course everyone is different), but the philosophy and approach to chronic pain management should not really vary from patient to patient.

Acknowledgments

I will take this opportunity to give recognition to my deceased brilliant psychiatrist father, Harry P. Loomer, M.D., a Renaissance man who was a student of the legendary psychiatrist, Carl Jung in Zurich, Switzerland, many years ago.

Wholehearted and enormous thanks goes out to Lawrence A. Blake and Joan Moore Blake for their tireless and diligent input with the editing of the second edition of this book. They spent countless hours (long distance in Illinois), working on the book with me for well over a year. I am forever grateful for their time and dedication.

Finally, special thanks and appreciation goes out to Valerie Blake Koch. She was with me every step of the way from start to finish of the book. She inspired and motivated me to write the book, and her input through every facet of the production of this book was invaluable.

About The Author

Jeffrey B. Loomer, M.D., FACP, FACR, is a Board Certified Rheumatologist, who maintains a demanding private medical practice limited to the management of patients with connective tissue and chronic pain disorders. A large segment of his patient population suffers from fibromyalgia and other chronic painful conditions. His patient population base consists of people living in southern Arizona and some of the surrounding states. He has been in solo private practice in Tucson, Arizona since 1992.

Dr. Loomer received his Bachelor of Science Degree from the State University of New York College at Oneonta. He holds a Master of Science Degree in Biomedical Sciences from Barry University in Miami Shores, Florida. Dr. Loomer graduated from St. George's University School of Medicine in Grenada, West Indies. He completed an Internal Medicine Internship at Greater Baltimore Medical Center in Baltimore, Maryland and an Internal Medicine Residency at New Britain General Hospital in New Britain, Connecticut. He then went on to complete a two year Rheumatology Fellowship at Dartmouth-Hitchcock Medical Center in Hanover, New Hampshire.

Dr. Loomer is a Fellow of the American College of Rheumatology and a Fellow of the American College of Physicians. Throughout the years, he has been involved with medical education in several different capacities. He was a Clinical Instructor in Medicine at Dartmouth Medical School, Medical House Staff Lecturer at Tucson General Hospital, Question Writer for the American Board of Internal Medicine Certification Examination, Peer Review Case Consultant for the Arizona Board of Medical Examiners, Admissions Committee Interviewer for The University of Arizona School of Medicine and has participated on Medical Advisory Panels to several pharmaceutical companies. In addition, Dr. Loomer has given many lectures on fibromyalgia, chronic pain and other rheumatologic conditions to physician groups in Tucson, Phoenix and New Mexico, as well as, local community based general public venues.

Dr. Loomer has also worked with The American College of Rheumatology as a Congressional Patient Advocate Delegate in Washington, D.C.

Author's Note

Dr. Loomer is available for speaking engagements and book signing events.

Inquiries should be e-mailed to mysterydocpublishing@gmail.com

Available from Amazon.com, fibromyalgiachronicpain.tripod.com, and other retail outlets

http://fibromyalgiachronicpain.tripod.com

It is available as an e-book from the following sites:
E-book: Amazon, iBooks, Barnes & Noble, Sony and other devices

22841241R00149

Made in the USA
Middletown, DE
15 August 2015